FIT IN ONE YEAR

YURIY OLIYNYK DPT, CSCS, PES

ISBN-13: 9798607917173

I would like to dedicate this book to my wonderful kids **Diana** and **Daniel**

bigandstrongapp@gmail.com
www.bigandstrongapp.com
@bigandstrongapp

Table of Contents

WHY?

Ever since I was a little kid I was in love with exercise. It taught me discipline. It taught me patience. It taught me persistence. It kept me away from drugs. It gave me an outlet for stress relief. The list goes on and on.

But the older I get the more I realize that I am an oddball. Very few people feel the same way about exercise and they are already gym rats or involved in competitive sports. But then there is the rest of the population. The overwhelming majority. People who view exercising as a chore. People who dread it. Always looking for excuses to skip it.

Just think about this for a moment: people would rather sign up for bariatric surgeries than go for a walk a few times a week. An overweight young woman who had enough willpower to get through years and years of rigorous schooling to become a cardiologist cannot stick to a simple exercise routine for more than a month. A man who is prepared to work 60-70 hours a week to become a partner at a law firm will not find 30 minutes for gym even after his doctor tells him that he is reaching the point of diabetes and hypertension. How does this happen? It doesn't make any sense!

At first glance, it might appear that we are a nation obsessed with fitness. Professional athletes are making millions of dollars. Magazines are packed with "detoxifying" cleanses. Instagram feed is full of videos of girls exercising (some recorded from angles that could rival Kamasutra). Everyone is dressed in sportswear. Everyone is carrying water bottles. Seems that we are on the right track.

But let's dig a little deeper. How compatible is our culture with a healthy lifestyle? Let's look at some of the western traditions: Memorial Day, Thanksgiving, Christmas, birthdays, etc. What do they have in common? Easy – eating and drinking. None of them involve any physical activity. We don't reserve weekends for hiking with our family or Friday nights for breaking a sweat at the gym with our friends.

My point is that, unless you are already a part of the exercising community, a significant paradigm shift will be needed for you to make changes. It will not be easy and you will be swimming against the current. No surprise most people attempting to become fit inevitably fail. Get crushed by lifestyles not conducive to regular training schedules. Sabotaged by subconscious agendas of their friends and families.

Only those with the strongest character will be able to follow through while facing these obstacles. Are you one of them? Well, let's reflect for a moment: what thoughts this conversation has provoked in your head so far? Are you excited by the challenge or looking for a way out already? Are you humble enough to admit that some of this could apply to you or are you bored and irritated? You decide which way this is going to go. And there is a chance that you have made that decision already.

For a long time I've been puzzled by the whole notion of compliance with training. I've read a lot of smart books about different models of how to increase adherence. How to determine what stage the person is in. Identify the barriers. Develop appropriate strategies. Blah, blah, blah...

I have never seen any of it work. Never! People who are already fit somehow always manage to find their way to the gym. While people who are out of shape will have "legitimate" reasons to skip training every single day. These are usually the people who are also overweight because of the "bad metabolism." What a coincidence!

When you talk to people in the latter category, no matter what motivational speeches or rationale for exercising you give them, they will always find a reason why it is not going to happen. It seems that after decades of reality TV and talk shows we have become so good at rationalizing our BS that there is almost no way to get through. We are constantly reminded that it is ok to choose the path of the least resistance. Instead of embracing hard work, victim mentality is currently glorified.

But after observing all this for many years I started recognizing a pattern. I realized that people with poor compliance with training can be roughly grouped in one of the three stages. Similar to stages of grief. And to help you determine what stage you might fall into, each stage will have a catchphrase attached to it.

Stage one: "I don't care"

This one is not as obvious as you might think. Because most educated people are aware that we are *supposed* to care and not many of them will openly admit that they don't. That's why a better question to ask yourself is "WHY do I care?"

When it comes to exercising, there are three primary reasons for WHY you should care about this. Let's see if any of them can give you a sufficient WHY to make exercise a permanent part of your schedule for the rest of your life.

1. **Health benefits.** This might seem pretty straightforward but at the same time, it is not. Because outside of medical professionals very few people really understand what the link between exercising and your health is. And it's not uncommon for people to say something like "my grandma is 87 and she has never exercised, so I don't know what you are talking about."

2. **Athletic performance.** This one should be a little more obvious. There are very few jobs these days that actually require you to be fit. So unless you are a firefighter or in the military, physical fitness is not a major concern. And that's why it is completely acceptable for a young guy nowadays not to be able to do a single Pull-Up or even a Push-Up.

3. **Appearance.** Seems that we finally found one that actually matters and a lot of it has to do with making yourself appealing to the opposite gender. But even in this area there are plenty of shortcuts. Guys figured out that if you are good at banter and have a nice car, nobody will notice that you look like you are 7 months pregnant. Girls realized that as long as you are still young you will have plenty of options, despite being "curvy." On top of that, we are constantly being told to love our bodies the way they are. So who needs the gym? Must be for insecure or shallow people. "Get a life already!"

Stage two: "I don't have time"

These are the people who feel that they *should* care about this but are not disciplined enough to actually do it. But, of course, nobody wants to admit that. So what do you do? You keep repeating the same excuse over and over again until you start to believe in it yourself.

I was talking to my coworker a few years ago about my training and at some point during the conversation she said something like "I wish I had time to exercise." And it got me very curious because it was difficult for me to imagine that her schedule was busier than mine. So I started asking questions (I didn't know any better at that time). "Well, I have to walk my dog when I get home." But what if you do this? "Well, my friend doesn't want to go on those days." But what if you do that? "Well, the parking is bad."

And after we went back and forth for a few minutes I finally realized that theoretically, she would like to be in shape. But as long as she doesn't have to do absolutely anything. Which probably explains the popularity of various fitness gadgets. For example, you can just wear a watch that calculates your steps and feel like you are doing something without actually doing anything.

If you are reading this at home and do sincerely believe that you don't have time to exercise, put this book aside and do Burpees for five minutes in a row (if you are in decent shape you should get around 100). After that, it should become pretty obvious that getting a little exercise in your life is not a matter of a lot of time or some expensive equipment.

It is the norm for us to spend around 40 hours a week at our jobs because we all need money to live good lives. But if you think about it, the state of your health and fitness also has a significant effect on the quality of your life. And that is why three one hour training sessions a week should probably be considered a more or less permanent part of your weekly schedule and not just something that happens before weddings or vacations in tropical countries.

Stage three: "At least I try"

These are usually the people who *want* the benefits of exercising but only as long as it doesn't require too much effort. For some, the price they are not willing to pay might be the actual workout, for others – learning about working out properly. Let's look at a couple of examples.

A married woman with two kids made a New Year's resolution to get in shape. But now it is time to actually do it. Sigh. Well, her husband is not really in shape. So why does she need to look good for him? Plus she had two kids so nobody can judge her (although the kids are old already, but still...).

Unfortunately, she already told her friends about doing it and now she doesn't want them to think that she is lazy. Sigh. So she shows up at the gym without any idea of what she is supposed to do. Wanders around a bit, texts some friends, takes a selfie and goes home. And of course after about a month of doing that without getting any results whatsoever, she quits while feeling good about herself. "At least I tried."

Now let's look at a young guy. He actually doesn't mind going to the gym. His friends are there. Some pretty girls show up every once in a while. He loves gym! But you better not give him any books about training. Or tell him that the way he does a particular exercise is incredibly dangerous.

It seems that guys put knowing how to lift weights into the same macho category as knowing how to fight or knowing what to do in the bedroom. Meaning that no guy will ever admit that this is something he doesn't know anything about. So, instead, they just go to the gym and fake competence. And they will stick to their stubborn ways even if it leads to an injury. "At least I tried" (but with a deeper voice).

The bottom line

I am not trying to shame anyone or pass judgment here. All this discussion is meant to do is to help you make an honest assessment of where you stand in regards to exercise. And the fact that you are reading this book doesn't automatically absolve you. Find the real reason why you are out of shape. It is probably not because you don't have time or because exercise doesn't work for your "unique physiology."

If someone gave you a million dollars every time you came to the gym - you would show up every single time (probably would come early too). If someone gave you a billion dollars for learning the material presented in this book – you would memorize it from cover to cover. You wouldn't keep putting off reading it or quit halfway because "it's complicated."

My point is that if this was important to you, you would get it done. And if it isn't, there is no way for me to trick you into wanting it. We all have different values. Some people love to cook, some people can't stand it. Similarly, some people love to exercise, while others hate it.

I don't want to get overly spiritual, but you are going to have to do some soul searching to find your WHY. It doesn't have to be very sophisticated and you don't need to reveal to anyone what it is. You want your ex-boyfriend's jaw to drop when you "accidentally" bump into him in a year – I love it! You want to get in shape so you can get out of your parent's basement and enlist in the military – I salute you!

Whatever your WHY is, it just has to be strong enough. Strong enough for you to learn the system presented in this book, even if you have to read it ten times. Strong enough not to skip a training session just because you got held up at work. Even if it's late. Even if it's snowing outside. Three times a week. For the next twelve months.

OVERVIEW

First thing first

This system is written for relatively healthy adults but I can't assume that that's everyone who decides to read this book. And having a long history of prior inactivity does not shift the odds in your favor. Which means that you have to see a doctor before getting started. Bring this book with you and ask if this system is appropriate for you considering your age and medical history. Any cardiac or orthopedic conditions you might have, need to be discussed in detail.

Another major concern is being severely overweight. I do believe that it is possible to get in shape in a year but we also have to be realistic. If you weigh double of what is appropriate for your height – you are starting out in a hole.

The system presented in this book is designed to help you to get started from a complete zero. But if you carry a few hundred pounds of extra weight - you might need some work just to get to zero. Ask your doctor if you can start doing some walking on a regular basis. Have him or her set you up with a dietician. And be patient. You probably gained all that weight over the course of many years. So don't expect to get rid of it in just a few weeks.

Proper nutrition is as important for being fit and healthy as training. You can't compensate for slacking with your diet by doing well at the gym. Nutrition overview presented later in this book, however, is there just to give you a general outline. I will not be sufficient for people with eating disorders. If there is a chance that you might be in that category – seek professional counseling.

Too many options

I've trained with some of the most elite military units and at some of the best martial arts gyms in the world. I do know that there are many ways to get in shape. You could do battle ropes, swing kettlebells, hit a punching bag, run hills, flip tires, etc. There are hundreds of other exercises and every time I open social media I see a new "functional" movement being invented.

But at the end of the day, we have to decide on what you are actually going to do. How to cover all the bases without spending an unreasonable amount of time training? What equipment an average gym will have available? What drills are overly complicated for someone to be able to learn without a coach? What movements are too dangerous and should be left for professionals?

Once you start considering all these factors, your options become much narrower. In reality, all we need is a few basic exercises to target major muscle groups and some cardio on top of it. Remember, this book is about becoming a well-rounded athlete and making you look like one. So don't be surprised that there are no triceps Pushdowns or any other fluff included.

It is interesting how conversations about working out usually tend to turn into purely theoretical discussions. People who don't have access to a pool talk about how beneficial swimming is. Guys who are too lazy to go for a walk a couple of times a week tell me how they wish they could learn Muay Thai. Seems that the only muscles people are willing to exercise these days are their tongues.

Our agenda is different. Instead of just talking about becoming fit we will focus on how to actually make it happen. How to turn someone with zero training experience into a badass. So you can look at yourself in the mirror a year from now and be blown away by how far you have come.

Throughout this book I will insist that you follow its precise recommendations. But that's not because I enjoy telling people what to do. There will always be those who just have to learn from their own mistakes. No matter what logic you present them with for why there is an optimum way to do something, they will do the very opposite just so they don't feel like their freedoms are violated. Or maybe they really do know something about training that I don't. It is not impossible. All I am saying is that if you came to me and asked how to get in the best shape of your life in the fastest way possible, I would tell you exactly what is written in this book.

If you are completely new to this, the description of this training system might seem very complicated at first. Don't let it overwhelm you. Once you start actually doing it you will see that it is as straightforward as it gets. Also, you do not have to read the whole book at once. Finish the level that you are about to start and read the description of the following level when it is time for you to move up.

Overall structure

Unwillingness to learn about proper training methodology is a sure sign of the eventual failure when it comes to exercising. A lot of it has to do with the level of maturity: if you understand that physical training in one form or another should be a part of your routine for the rest of your life, then reading a few pages about how to do it correctly won't seem like too much to ask. Did you obsess about your feelings when you were learning how to drive? Did you quit because "it wasn't fun"? Perhaps you could adopt a similar businesslike attitude towards learning about training (and subsequently training itself). Here we go.

All training programs presented in this book prescribe three training sessions a week scheduled on nonconsecutive days. Stick to it. Some people get overly motivated and decide to train every day. But keep in mind that training is only one side of the equation and it has to be balanced out with proper nutrition and plenty of sleep. If you don't get enough rest between your training sessions the fatigue will accumulate and over time might result in **overtraining**. Think of training as sun tanning and overtraining as a sunburn. Not only will a sunburn (overtraining) undo all your work, but now you will also have to give your body time to heal before going back to sun tanning (training) again.

If you want to stay active on the days you don't have gym – go for a walk. You can walk for one hour, two hours or even more. As long as your joints are ok with it. You can also do some stretching combined with foam rolling on those days. This is a great way to speed up the recovery and prevent injuries. But stay away from the gym! Once you start lifting relatively heavy weights and reach decent running speed, three training sessions a week will no longer seem insufficient.

This system is set in four stages (levels). You will spend 12 weeks in each level with a week of rest in between:

Weeks 1-12: Level 1, week 13: rest;
Weeks 14-25: Level 2, week 26: rest;
Weeks 27-38: Level 3, week 39: rest;
Weeks 40-51: Level 4, week 52: rest.

Each successive level will be more difficult than the previous one. Keep that in mind before moving forward. For example, if you feel that the level you are currently in is just right – stay in it. Not everybody wants to be an Olympic caliber athlete or to train as hard as one. It is better to find the level that fits your goals and make it a habit for the rest of your life rather than pushing yourself just to prove a point and then end up quitting training altogether.

If you have some prior experience with training similar to what is presented here, you can start at the level that is more appropriate. But don't fool yourself. If you have never read a single book about resistance training, you can roam around the gym for many years and still be a complete beginner. And knowing that Dumbbell Curls are for biceps and Bench Press is for chest doesn't change anything. Swallow your ego and start at Level 1.

Week of rest between levels does not necessarily mean that you shouldn't train at all. Prolonged rest break will signal to your body that increased level of physical fitness is no longer required and will lead to regression of performance (**detraining**). As a result, when you finally return to training it might feel like you starting from a complete zero again.

That's why, although it is not unheard of to take a complete week off from training here and there, a smarter way to go about it is to decrease your training to the point where it feels like rest while doing just enough to prevent detraining. Such periods are called **deloads** and people who do not see the need in them usually don't train very hard to begin with.

You will have two options for your deloads. Option one is the minimum I want you to do. Option two is the maximum I want you to do. If you feel slightly burned out and in need of a break – go with option one. On the other hand, if you feel on a roll and want to keep going – pick option two.

The intensity level for your deload weeks will be based on your performance during your last training session of a particular level. Regardless of what level you are in, deloads will stay about the same and will resemble Level 1 training sessions. That is why the descriptions of the two deload options presented below will make more sense once you are already familiar with the Level 1 program.

1st deload option:

- You will train only once during that week (preferably somewhere in the middle).
- You will only do the first set in all resistance exercises (first warm-up).
- In Back Extensions and Sit-Ups, you will do about half of the reps from what you were able to do in your last session.
- You will only do one round of running (reduce the speed to whatever feels comfortable).

2nd deload option:

- You will train twice during that week.
- You will only do the first two sets in all resistance exercises (first and second warm-ups).
- In Back Extensions and Sit-Ups, you will do about two-thirds of the reps from what you were able to do in your last session prior to deload.
- You will only do two rounds of running (reduce the speed to whatever feels comfortable).

Once again: even when you reach higher levels your deload weeks will still be one of the above options (and not based on whatever program you are currently using). The only difference will be that later on you might be using slightly heavier weights and higher running speed during your deloads. But don't get overzealous. Remember these weeks are about active rest.

It is better to schedule deloads during weeks when you know it will be difficult to train. For example, when you covering nights at the hospital or taking your kids on vacation. Some levels might have to be scheduled for 10 weeks, others – for 14. And even if you plan ahead, things will not always go as expected. Those who have a genuine WHY will find a way to make it work, those who don't – will find an excuse to quit.

Regardless of whether you decided to take a complete week off from training or did deload as prescribed, do not expect to show up on the first day of the following level and start with the same weights and running speed you were able to do at your previous peak. That would not be a wise strategy even if you did retain your top level of performance. A smarter approach would be to take a few steps back and slowly get back to your best over a few weeks. This will give your body a chance to get back in the groove and create some momentum before making a leap ahead. Treat your body fairly and it will cooperate. Get pushy and impatient and it will rebel, after which any further progress will become an uphill battle.

Reps and sets

Lifting a load up and down one time is considered a repetition (*rep*). Raising the load up is called concentric portion of the rep. Lowering it down – eccentric portion. The speed ("tempo") of each portion can vary depending on the mode of training. Bodybuilding style of training usually dictates slower speed – about two seconds for each portion. In strength training concentric phase is much more explosive, which allows heavier loads to be lifted. For our purposes, however, we are not going to get too technical here. Just make sure to complete each rep through a full range of motion (ROM) in a smooth controlled manner.

Performing a few repetitions in a row without breaks is called a set of repetitions (*set*). When training load is selected for a set it is usually estimated that the maximum number of reps it can be lifted (before fatiguing) will fall within a particular range. The desired number of repetitions per set will vary based on the goal. 1-6 reps are considered to be the best for strength development. 6-12 are the best for increasing muscle size. 15 reps or higher are considered to be endurance work. Which is not to say that sets of 1 to 6 reps will not make you any bigger or doing 12 to 6 reps will not make you any stronger. Obviously, there is at least some overlap.

Sets are divided into warm-up sets (described later) and work sets. Work sets are considered to be the sets in which you are handling the main training load (MTL) assigned for that session. The number of work sets per exercise is normally from 1 to 5. If the same load is being used for all work sets, they are referred to as *sets across*. If the load is increased from one work set to another, it is called a *pyramid*.

There are different ways to record sets and reps. For the purpose of this book the first number will be the sets and what follows after "x" will apply to reps. For example, 3x10 means three sets of ten reps.

The rest between sets will depend on the training mode of the session. During strength work, long rest breaks (up to 5 minutes) are normally practiced. During hypertrophy sessions, the rest breaks are kept shorter (around a minute) in order to maintain muscle "pump" from set to set. For the endurance training, rest breaks are kept to 30 seconds or less and sometimes different exercises are rotated without any rest in between (*circuit training*).

The amount of rest between sets will also depend on the exercise itself. For example, you will need more rest between sets of Squats than between sets of Shoulder Press. On occasion, very heavy sets of Deadlifts and Squats might require rest breaks even longer than 5 minutes. In this case, an effort must be made to stay warm and mentally focused.

Warm-up

There are two types of warm-up: general and specific. General warm-up is an activity performed at the beginning of a training session designed to get your mind and body ready for the following work. This activity should not be too strenuous. For example, five minutes of jump rope (if you are lighter) or stationary bike (if you are heavier).

General warm-up will be the only optional part of training sessions. So, for example, if you live in Texas and your gym doesn't have an air conditioner, you might feel warm enough to get started just from walking from your car. With that being said, do understand that the older you get the more important general warm-up will become.

A specific warm-up is done for every exercise individually. These are going to be all of the sets leading to the work sets. Their purpose is to get you ready for the following hard work. During Levels 1 and 2 all sets except the very last one will be considered warm-ups. For example, if you are planning to do Bench Press with 40-pound dumbbells as your MTL for 10 reps, the warm-up could be the following:

20s for 10 reps;
30s for 10 reps.

These are some of the general guidelines in regards to warm-up sets:

- The colder it is at the gym, the more warm-up you will need.

- The more difficult exercises will generally require more warm-up than the easier ones. For example, you will probably need more warm-up sets for Squats than for Pulldowns.

- The exercises that are earlier in your workout will normally require more sets than the later ones. For example, by the time you reach Back Extensions and Sit-Ups you are probably not going to need any warm-up sets at all.

- The more advanced you get the more warm-up you will probably require. It takes more time to get ready to Deadlift 750 pounds than 75.

- Training sessions with lower reps will generally require more warm-up sets than training sessions with higher reps. Naturally, when you are doing Squats for 3x5 you will use a lot heavier weight than if you did 3x10. Therefore, in the former training session, you would need more time to warm-up than in the latter.

- Straps and weightlifting belts should not be used during warm-up sets (with exception of some special circumstances).

- Stay active during the warm-up: massage any tender spots, address any areas that require additional attention (rotator cuff, hip mobility), etc.

Stretching

Every training session should end with some stretching. Learning how to properly stretch might not be as easy as it seems. Developing the ability to relax the muscle while stretching it will take some time. It is not "no pain, no gain" here. Static stretch positions are held for 20-30 seconds while slowly increasing the ROM. If the stretch is unilateral, don't forget to do it for both sides of the body. Also, remember not to hold your breath while performing stretching.

The stretches I listed later in this book are the bare minimum. The reason I did not prescribe more, is because that could extend your session quite a bit. But if you want to add a few – feel free to do so. This portion of the training session can be pretty flexible (literally and figuratively).

Main muscle groups

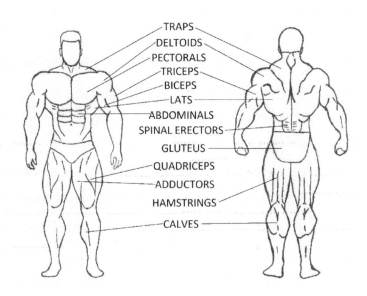

Don't be a hero

If you have never trained before, make sure to start with very light weights and give yourself plenty of time to learn the proper form for all exercises. It will usually take at least a few weeks. Being impatient and careless during this time can turn a healthy exercise habit into an ultimate catastrophe.

It is important to understand that participation in any vigorous physical activity involves the risk of a potential injury. And it is your responsibility to take every precaution to reduce your chances of getting hurt. Sufficient warm-up and proper technique are a big part of that. But there are also many other ways to screw up.

For example, I did not feel like bothering with safety collars during barbell exercises until I had plates rolling off on one side during Squats. I did not think that using a "thumbless" grip (thumbs are on the same side as the rest of the fingers) during Bench Press was that big of a deal until the bar slipped out of my hands and crashed into my chest. Luckily both of those instances happened during warm-up sets and did not cause a significant injury.

Another important, but often overlooked, aspect of training is that injuries do not happen only during the actual exercise execution. Awkward body mechanics while getting into starting position and returning the weight could put you at greater risk than the exercise itself.

When I write instructions for all the exercises presented later in this book I don't expect you to do something that generally resembles them. No! I expect you to do exactly what it says. Attention to detail here is everything. If you are very uncoordinated it might be a good idea to hire a personal trainer for a few weeks to help you learn all the exercises. Just be wary of them hitting you with limited-time-offer-lowest-price-ever deals and try to sign you up as a permanent client. To say that they are not cheap is an understatement.

Pay attention to developing rhythmical breathing patterns while learning new exercises. Compound movements that involve stabilization of torso might require a brief holding of breath while getting through "sticking" points, especially when heavy loads are used. However, care must be taken to make sure that this is not done excessively, as such practices put a lot of strain on the cardiovascular system.

Also, remember that no exercise should be causing excruciating pain. Because if it does – stop and assess the situation. Either you are performing it incorrectly or there is an underlying pathology that needs to be checked out by a qualified healthcare professional. In either case, don't wait for things to get worse and take the appropriate measures right away. Over time you will be able to tell the difference between discomfort in your muscles caused by hard work and the pain indicating that something is wrong.

LEVEL 1

There are two main prerequisites for you to be able to get started: you got a green light from your doctor and you have your WHY. Even if you are very motivated the first few sessions will feel like an uphill battle. You have to adjust your daily routine to schedule regular training sessions. You have to find a gym and what to wear. You have to learn all the exercises while feeling like everyone around is watching (or even laughing at you). The whole time your overprotective mind is going to keep producing "legitimate" reasons for why should quit: they should accept you the way you are, you don't have to prove anything to anyone, you are going to get injured...

At times like that, it will be imperative for you to remember WHY you are doing this. If you ever rode a bike, you know that the first few yards are always the hardest - it takes some effort to gain momentum. But once you have reached the desired speed, maintaining it is pretty easy. The same thing happens with working out – once you get past the initial frustration, continuing to exercise will be pretty easy.

The description of this training program might seem a bit rudimentary and could tempt you to skip forward to a more "serious" level. Don't! When you just start training your main goal is to learn the proper techniques of exercises. To make this process easier it is best to focus only on the few main moves and not make things overly complicated. The reason why I "spell everything out" is because I assume that whoever is reading this doesn't know anything about training.

MONDAY	WEDNESDAY	FRIDAY
Goblet squat 3x10	Goblet squat 3x10	Goblet squat 3x10
Lunge 3x(5+5)	Lunge 3x(5+5)	Lunge 3x(5+5)
Dumbbell bench press 3x10	Dumbbell bench press 3x10	Dumbbell bench press 3x10
Standing dumbbell shoulder press 3x10	Standing dumbbell shoulder press 3x10	Standing dumbbell shoulder press 3x10
Pulldowns 3x10	Pulldowns 3x10	Pulldowns 3x10
Seated cable row 3x10	Seated cable row 3x10	Seated cable row 3x10
Back extension 1xAMRAP	Back extension 1xAMRAP	Back extension 1xAMRAP
Sit-up 1xAMRAP	Sit-up 1xAMRAP	Sit-up 1xAMRAP
Running 3X3 min	Running 3X3 min	Running 3X3 min

In the first six exercises, you will be doing 3 sets of 10 reps (3x10) while using a pyramid method. You will be resting about a minute or two between each set. I have basic exercise tutorials posted on my "Big and Strong" YouTube channel. All of them are purposely designed to be 1 to 2 minutes. So you can review them between sets while keeping an appropriate pace.

In the first set, you will be using the weight that is approximately 50% of what you are planning to use in the last set. In the second set, you will be using the weight that is approximately 75% of what you are planning to use in the last set. The weight that you are using in the third set will be considered MTL. For example, if you are planning to use 20 pounds in your last set of Goblet Squat, your session could look like this:

1st set: 10lbs 10 reps (warm-up)

2nd set: 15lbs 10 reps (warm-up)

3rd set: 20lbs 10 reps (work set)

Don't get overly hung up on all the numbers during your first few training sessions. Just start with a very small weight and focus on the technique. If your form looks good, try slightly heavier weight for the following set. Then repeat it once again if everything goes well.

If, on the other hand, your technique in the second set started to deteriorate – stop after two sets and move on to the following exercise. Remember, we are not trying to set a new world record here. As I said many times already, your priority is learning the proper form. Faulty patterns learned in the initial stages of training are very difficult to correct later on. Another reason to be prudent during the first few training sessions is to avoid unnecessarily severe muscle soreness during the following days.

After you are done with the first six exercises, you will rest a minute or two and perform a set of Back Extensions and Sit-Ups. In each exercise, you will do as many reps as possible (AMRAP). Once again, rest for a minute or two and we are off to the running.

I prefer to use the treadmill because it is easier to control all of the parameters. We will be using a 3 to 1 ratio. That means you will run for three minutes and then walk for one. You will repeat that for a total of three rounds.

It will take some experimentation to find what running speed is comfortable for you to start with. As always, it is better to start too easy than too hard. That speed will stay the same for all three rounds for that session. For the minute-long active rest periods between the rounds of running, you will use comfortable walking speed. Somewhere around 3 mph should be about right and it does not have to increase over time.

That's the whole training session and it should probably take you less than one hour. Now just add some stretching and you are done for the day. It might not appear all that difficult at first, but we are just getting started. Once your technique in all exercises stabilizes and you start becoming comfortable at the gym – the real work will begin.

Progression

In order for you to keep improving from session to session, your training sessions will have to become more challenging over time. This is called a principle of **progressive overload**. A few different means of progressive overload will be utilized in this training program.

For the first six exercises, we will be focusing on increasing the MTL used. We are going to continue to use Goblet Squat for illustration. Let's say you were able to complete 10 reps with 20 pounds during your first training session. If 20 pounds felt easy, for the following training session you could attempt 30. Let's say you were able to complete 10 reps again but this time it felt quite challenging. That means that it would probably be reasonable for you to move up only by 5 pounds next time.

Let's say you used 35 pounds during the next training session and were able to get 8 good Squats. That means that for the following training session you are staying with 35-pound dumbbell once again. Only when you are able to complete all ten reps with the weight you are currently using you have the green light to move up again. Also, keep in mind that the reps that were performed with improper technique or required assistance from your training partner are not to be counted.

When you are increasing the weight you are using in your last set of a particular exercise make sure to adjust your warmups as well. It will not always be exactly 50% and 75%, but try to stay somewhere close to those guidelines. Also, take into account that during Squats and Lunges your bodyweight is a big part of the total load lifted. So you can slightly adjust the percentages because of that. But don't complicate things too much. Keep it simple: two progressively heavier warm-ups, plus one work set.

When it comes to Back Extensions and Sit-Ups you will be focusing on increasing the number of the reps performed. Try to beat whatever number you completed last time by at least one rep. If the number of reps becoming very high, add a little more resistance at the next session. Grab a plate and hold it over your chest with your arms crossed. This will initially decrease your reps count and you will have to work your way up again.

For running you will focus on increasing the speed. If you started with 4 mph and were able to complete 3 three minute rounds without overexerting yourself, you can move up to 4.1 next time. Once you have reached the speed with which you couldn't finish all 3 rounds you will stay with it until you are able to do it.

Hopefully, the above illustration made it clear how beneficial the training log is. It is very difficult to remember all weights, reps and speed for every exercise. An accurate training log will allow you to see how you are progressing from session to session, week to week and month to month. My "Big and Strong" app can help you keep records.

Patience

It is important to be patient when you are implementing progressive overload. Remember, the purpose of a training session is to provide stimulus to which your body has to respond. Numerous adaptations have to take place and it will require time and proper nutrition. Any attempts to force this process will probably lead to deterioration of technique, injuries and overtraining.

Let's imagine that during your first training session you used a 25-pound dumbbell for your Goblet Squat. You keep focusing on technique and add only 5 pounds from session to session. That would mean that you increase your Squat by 15 pounds every week and by the end of week 12 (theoretically) could reach 200. If you have ever seen a 200-pound dumbbell – you know that that would be quite an achievement.

The point is that there is no need to rush. Remember the story of the Tortoise and the Hare. Small consistent improvements will lead to huge gains over time. While being impatient and unreasonable might just put you in the "At least I try" stage discussed in the first chapter.

Modifications

As I write these training programs, I am not secretly hoping that guys will figure out to add Biceps Curls somewhere and ladies realize that I forgot about Hip Thrust. There are no hidden messages in the text or secret VIP-only versions of this program. What is written here is exactly what I think is the very best. So stop telling yourself how special you are and stick to the plan. Unless you are working around an injury or a disability, only the following modifications could be considered:

1. If you find that even bodyweight Squats and Lunges are too difficult for you to start with, temporarily substitute them with Leg Press to get your legs a little stronger.
2. Those who are able to perform Pull-Ups can use them instead of Pulldowns (while using additional weight as a form of progression). Kipping Pull-Ups, however, should not be considered as an alternative.
3. If you can't do Back Extensions properly initially, skip them completely for a while and attempt again a month or two later.
4. If you find that Sit-Ups are too difficult for you early on, substitute them with Crunches and go back to Sit-Ups when you are ready.
5. Even if you got cleared by your doctor to use this training program but find yourself significantly overweight, it might be wise to do walking instead of running initially. Start with whatever distance is comfortable and slowly increase it over time. Once you have lost a sufficient amount of weight, you can start running while using the method described earlier.

LEVEL 2

The main condition for you to be able to move up to this level is that by now your technique in all exercises is perfect. Another requirement is that by this point you are already running. Meaning that if you still use walking as a substitute because you are too heavy - you are not ready. Don't feel bad about it. You are on the right track. So what if it's going to take you a few extra months? Look on the bright side: the ultimate transformation is going to be much more drastic than if you were in a decent shape to begin with. Just don't forget to take some "before" pictures.

You will notice that training methodology becomes increasingly more complex with each successive level. It is a logical progression that is necessary to keep improving you as an athlete. It is also understandable how things can start getting a bit confusing for people with no prior exercise experience. In a way, it is expected. Think about it. If someone who does not know anything about Jiu-Jitsu went straight to a black belt class, chances are that person would have no idea what was going on. Regardless of how intelligent or well-educated he or she is.

The same thing with resistance training. Only instead of a belt system, we will use levels. Remember, they are designed to build upon each other. That is why I stated earlier in this book that you do not have to read it all at once. It is easier to make sense of each following level after you spend three months familiarizing yourself with the previous one. But go with whichever way of reading makes more sense to you.

If you just finished Level 1 and it is time for you to move up – congratulations! Consider yourself a "blue belt" of resistance training. Towards the end of Level 1, you might have noticed that you are not progressing as fast as in the beginning. The reason for that is **accommodation**. Your body is getting used to the training stress it is subjected to and no longer needs to produce a significant adaptation. Which is why the rate of your progress at the gym decreases over time.

In order to avoid accommodation, at this point we are going to introduce **variation**. And we are going to accomplish this by making training sessions of the same week slightly different from each other:

MONDAY - A	WEDNESDAY - B	FRIDAY - C
Back squat 5x5	Back squat 4x10	Back squat 3x15
Lunge 5x(5+5)	Lunge 4x(10+10)	Lunge 3x(15+15)
Barbell bench press 5x5	Barbell bench press 4x10	Barbell bench press 3x15
Standing dumbbell shoulder press 5x5	Standing dumbbell shoulder press 4x10	Standing dumbbell shoulder press 3x15
Pulldowns 5x5	Pulldowns 4x10	Pulldowns 3x15
Seated cable row 5x5	Seated cable row 4x10	Seated cable row 3x15
Back extension 1xAMRAP	Back extension 1xAMRAP	Back extension 1xAMRAP
Sit-up 1xAMRAP	Sit-up 1xAMRAP	Sit-up 1xAMRAP
Running 3X3 min	Running 4X3 min	Running 5X3 min

You might have noticed that there are two new exercises listed in this program. First is the Back Squat instead of Goblet Squat. The reason I am making this substitution is because, as you might have noticed by now, once you start using heavier weight it becomes very difficult to hold it in your hands during Goblet Squat.

The second one is Barbell Bench Press instead of Dumbbell Bench Press. The reason here is very similar to the Squat: once you start using heavy dumbbells it becomes tricky to balance them or even to get them into starting position. Barbell solves both of those problems.

You might also have noticed that the prescribed number of sets and reps for the first six exercises is different for different days of the week. This is one of the very common ways to introduce variation into your training called *daily undulating periodization.*

On Mondays in the first six exercises, you will be performing 5 sets of 5 reps while using a pyramid scheme. That means that over five sets you will be working your way up to the heaviest weight that you can lift for 5 reps. For example, if you are planning to attempt 100 pounds for five reps, your session could look like this:

1st set – 5 reps with 40 pounds;
2nd set – 5 reps with 55 pounds;
3rd set – 5 reps with 70 pounds;
4th set – 5 reps with 85 pounds;
5th set – 5 reps with 100 pounds.

On Wednesdays in the first six exercises, you will be performing 4 sets of 10 reps while using a pyramid scheme. That means that over four sets you will be working your way up to the heaviest weight that you can lift for 10 reps. For example, if you are planning to attempt 80 pounds for ten reps, your session could look like this:

1st set – 10 reps with 35 pounds;
2nd set – 10 reps with 50 pounds;
3rd set – 10 reps with 65 pounds;
4th set – 10 reps with 80 pounds.

On Fridays in the first six exercises, you will be performing 3 sets of 15 reps while using a pyramid scheme. That means that over three sets you will be working your way up to the heaviest weight that you can lift for 15 reps. For example, if you are planning to attempt 60 pounds for fifteen reps, your session could look like this:

1st set – 15 reps with 40 pounds;
2nd set – 15 reps with 50 pounds;
3rd set – 15 reps with 60 pounds.

It should be obvious that the weight you are going to lift in the last set of a particular exercise on Monday will be heavier than the weight you will be lifting on Wednesday. And the weight you are going to lift in your last set on Wednesday will be heavier than the weight you will be lifting in that exercise on Friday.

Every week you will try to work up to a slightly heavier weight for a particular number of reps. Meaning that you will be comparing your performance on Monday to what you were able to do on the previous Monday, Wednesday to the previous Wednesday, and Friday to the previous Friday.

There are no longer exact percentages listed for the warm-up sets because at this point you should be able to estimate them. Also, the number of warm-ups will not always be the same as is prescribed for different days of the week. For example, if you are planning to do Lunges with 20-pound dumbbells for 5 reps in your last set, there is no need to drag it out over four warm-ups. Do one set with just bodyweight, one set with 10-pound dumbbells and go for the 20s in the next one.

On the other hand, if you worked your way up to 5 reps with 185 for your fifth set of Bench Press but it felt pretty easy - do an extra set and go for 190-195. Just don't use such flexibility to start favoring exercises that you like at the expense of the ones you don't like. Stick to the recommended template as your default and use general guidelines presented on page 15 to make adjustments.

You could also adjust rest breaks between sets on different days of the week. Since on Mondays we are trying to lift heavier loads you could rest 2 to 3 minutes between your sets. This workout will probably turn out to be the longest. On Wednesdays, we will stay with our usual 1 to 2 minutes. Finally, on Fridays, we will be focusing on endurance and will keep the rest breaks to 30-60 seconds.

For Back Extensions and Sit-Ups, we could introduce a little variety by doing the following. On Mondays in these two exercises, you would do AMRAP while holding 10-pound plate on your chest. On Wednesdays, you would do AMRAP while holding 5-pound plate on your chest. And on Fridays, you would do AMRAP without any additional weight.

It should be obvious that on Friday you should be able to complete more reps than you did on Wednesday. And on Wednesday you should be able to complete more reps than you did on Monday. Once again you will be comparing your performance on a particular day of the week to your performance on the same day of the week from the previous week.

Things will also be different for running. You will continue using a 3 to 1 ratio but the number of rounds you are completing will be different for different days of the week: on Monday you will do three rounds, on Wednesday – 4, and on Friday – 5. The speed of running will stay the same for a particular week.

For example, if you started with 6 mph and have gone through all three sessions, you will increase the speed by 0.1 mph and go back to 3x3, 4x3 and 5x3. When that's accomplished you'll go up to 6.2 and go through the rotation again. If you were unable to complete all prescribed rounds, you will stay with the same speed for the next week. Once again, the speed and duration of walking in between rounds stay constant from session to session and from week to week.

LEVEL 3

Level 3 training program is going to be a significant step up from Level 2. Take that into consideration before getting started. If you just want to be fit, Level 1 or Level 2 programs are completely fine. On the other hand, if you are a firefighter, police officer or in the military - Level 3 is just what you need.

At this point, the effort you exert in each exercise will become so great that it will be impractical to perform all of them in the same training session. That is why you will notice that training sessions of different days of the week do not contain the same exercises.

Odd Weeks

MONDAY – 1A	WEDNESDAY – 1B	FRIDAY – 1C
Back squat 3x5	Barbell bench press 3x5	Deadlift 3x5
EMOM: 1. Pulldown 5x10 2. Standing dumbbell shoulder press 5x10 3. Lunge 5x(5+5)	EMOM: 1. Seated cable row 5x10 2. Dumbbell bench press 5x10 3. Goblet squat 5x10	EMOM: 1. Pulldown 5x10 2. Standing dumbbell shoulder press 5x10 3. Lunge 5x(5+5)
Back extension 1xAMRAP	Sit-up 1xAMRAP	Back extension 1xAMRAP
Running 3x4 min	Running 4x4 min	Running 5x4 min

Even weeks

MONDAY – 2A	WEDNESDAY – 2B	FRIDAY – 2C
Back squat 3x5	Barbell bench press 3x5	Deadlift 3x5
EMOM: 1. Seated cable row 5x10 2. Dumbbell bench press 5x10 3. Goblet squat 5x10	EMOM: 1. Pulldown 5x10 2. Standing dumbbell shoulder press 5x10 3. Lunge 5x(5+5)	EMOM: 1. Seated cable row 5x10 2. Dumbbell bench press 5x10 3. Goblet squat 5x10
Sit-up 1xAMRAP	Back extension 1xAMRAP	Sit-up 1xAMRAP
Running 3x4 min	Running 4x4 min	Running 5x4 min

* warm-up sets are not listed

The first exercise of each session will be performed for 3 sets of 5 reps (not counting the warm-ups) while using a sets across scheme. We are going to use Squat to illustrate the progression. Let's say on Monday of week 1 you used 135lbs and were able to perform 3 sets of 5 reps. This means that for the following Monday you can increase the MTL for Squat by 5 or 10 pounds. Let's say you went up to 145 and were able to get 3x5 again. Then for the following Squat session, you can increase the weight by 5 to 10 pounds, once again. On Monday of the third week, you used 155, but this time were able to get only 5, 5, 4. This means that you should stay with that MTL for another training session.

Let's say that on Monday of week four you were able to complete 5 reps in all three sets. It is time to increase MTL again. On Monday of week five you went for 165 and got 5, 4, 3 reps. As you might have already guessed, we will be staying with 165 for another week. Let's say on Monday of week six you improve to 5, 5, 4 and on Monday of week seven, you finally get 3x5. You are now clear to go up in weight again. Use your discretion though. Since things are toughening up, maybe it would be reasonable to increase weight only by 5 pounds for the next Monday and go up to 170.

During the first exercise you will rest about 2 to 3 minutes between each set. The pace will pick up after that as you will move on to the EMOM rotations. Chances are you will not need much of an additional warm-up while transitioning from strength exercises to these rotations. All I usually do is 10 Push-Ups on Monday and Friday and 10 bodyweight Squats on Wednesday.

EMOM stands for every minute on the minute. You will need some kind of timer to be able to stay on track. With this protocol, you perform one set of an exercise at the beginning of every minute. Once all the prescribed reps are completed, you will rest for the remaining time of that minute before moving on to the following exercise.

For example, once you have completed a set of Pulldowns you will rest the remaining time of that minute and then start a set of Standing Shoulder Press exactly at the beginning of the next minute. Once that set is completed, you will put the dumbbells down and rest the remaining time of the second minute. After which you will proceed to Lunges (five lunges on each leg) with the same weight you used for Shoulder Press. Once Lunges are completed and you rested the remaining time of the third minute, you will start a set of Pulldowns at the beginning of the fourth minute.

As you can see, that's three exercises performed for five sets of ten reps in a 15-minute period. This should make it obvious that the weights you will use during EMOM rotations won't be even close to the weights you were able to lift in those exercises for 10 reps during Level 2. Therefore, don't be too stingy with the weight reduction. Get used to this pace first and then start slowly increasing the weights you are using from session to session.

Instead of doing Back Extensions and Sit-Ups every time, you will now alternate them from session to session. When it comes to running, you will start using 4-minute rounds (heavier trainees can stay with three minutes). The speed will now vary for different days of the same week: on Wednesday you will use the speed that is 1 mph less than what you did on Monday, on Friday – 1 mph less than what you did on Wednesday. The speed will increase simultaneously for all sessions of the week:

	MONDAY	WEDNESDAY	FRIDAY
WEEK 1	3X4 (7 mph)	4x4 (6 mph)	5x4 (5 mph)
WEEK 2	3X4 (7.1 mph)	4x4 (6.1 mph)	5x4 (5.1 mph)
WEEK 3	3X4 (7.2 mph)	4x4 (6.2 mph)	5x4 (5.2 mph)

For the meticulous types

For those who are more comfortable with the precise recommendations, I designed a system for calculating the number of warm-up sets for the strength exercises of Levels 3 and 4. Using this model is completely optional and most people will probably find the guidelines presented on page 15 more helpful.

The system is based on the assumption that the heavier the weight you are using in relation to your bodyweight the more warm-up sets you will need. Another factor we are taking into account is that in different exercises the same weight on the bar will present different degrees of challenge.

$$ k = \frac{MTL}{Bodyweight} $$

Once you divided the MTL you plan to use in a particular exercise by your bodyweight, find the number of the recommended warm-up sets in the table below. If the k you received during your calculations is lower than what is required for even one warm-up set for that particular exercise (which should probably not be the case at this level), then technically no warm-ups are prescribed. Obviously individual circumstances can override these guidelines while determining the exact prescription.

k	≥ 0.5	≥ 0.75	≥ 1	≥ 1.25	≥ 1.5	≥ 1.75	≥ 2
Bench	1	2	3	4	5		
Squat		1	2	3	4	5	
Deadlift			1	2	3	4	5

These are the recommended numbers of reps and approximate percentages of the loads for the warm-up sets based on the MTL planned to be used in the following work sets:

- 1 warm-up: 1st - 5 reps with 65% of MTL.
- 2 warm-ups: 1st - 5 reps with 50% of MTL; 2nd – 4 reps with 75% of MTL.
- 3 warm-ups: 1st – 5 reps with 40% of MTL; 2nd – 4 reps with 60% of MTL; 3rd – 3 reps with 80% of MTL.
- 4 warm-ups: 1st – 5 reps with 30% of MTL; 2nd – 4 reps with 47.5% of MTL; 3rd – 3 reps with 65% of MTL; 4th – 2 reps with 82.5% of MTL.
- 5 warm-ups: 1st – 5 reps with 25% of MTL; 2nd 4 reps with 40% of MTL; 3rd – 3 reps with 55% of MTL; 4th – 2 reps with 70% of MTL; 5th – 1 rep with 85% of MTL.

LEVEL 4

If you gave it all you got in the Level 3, by now you probably know that continued training at maximum capacity becomes increasingly difficult. That's why at some point variation of loading has to be implemented to avoid overtraining. That is the main difference between Level 4 and Level 3.

Week 1

MONDAY – 1A	WEDNESDAY – 1B	FRIDAY – 1C
Back squat 5x6 (80%)	Barbell bench press 5x6 (80%)	Deadlift 5x6 (80%)
CIRCUIT: 1. Pulldown 5x10 2. Standing dumbbell shoulder press 5x10 3. Lunge 5x(5+5)	CIRCUIT: 1. Seated cable row 5x10 2. Dumbbell bench press 5x10 3. Goblet squat 5x10	CIRCUIT: 1. Pulldown 5x10 2. Standing dumbbell shoulder press 5x10 3. Lunge 5x(5+5)
Back extension 1xAMRAP	Sit-up 1xAMRAP	Back extension 1xAMRAP
Running 3x5 min	Running 4x5 min	Running 5x5 min

Week 2

MONDAY – 2A	WEDNESDAY – 2B	FRIDAY – 2C
Back squat 5x4 (90%)	Barbell bench press 5x4 (90%)	Deadlift 5x4 (90%)
CIRCUIT: 1. Seated cable row 4x10 2. Dumbbell bench press 4x10 3. Goblet squat 4x10	CIRCUIT: 1. Pulldown 4x10 2. Standing dumbbell shoulder press 4x10 3. Lunge 4x(5+5)	CIRCUIT: 1. Seated cable row 4x10 2. Dumbbell bench press 4x10 3. Goblet squat 4x10
Sit-up 1xAMRAP	Back extension 1xAMRAP	Sit-up 1xAMRAP
Running 2x5 min	Running 3x5 min	Running 4x5 min

Week 3

MONDAY – 3A	WEDNESDAY – 3B	FRIDAY – 3C
Back squat 5x2 (100%)	Barbell bench press 5x2 (100%)	Deadlift 5x2 (100%)
CIRCUIT: 1. Pulldown 3x10 2. Standing dumbbell shoulder press 3x10 3. Lunge 3x(5+5)	CIRCUIT: 1. Seated cable row 3x10 2. Dumbbell bench press 3x10 3. Goblet squat 3x10	CIRCUIT: 1. Pulldown 3x10 2. Standing dumbbell shoulder press 3x10 3. Lunge 3x(5+5)
Back extension 1xAMRAP	Sit-up 1xAMRAP	Back extension 1xAMRAP
Running 1x5 min	Running 2x5 min	Running 3x5 min

* warm-up sets are not listed

During Level 4 we will be using *weekly undulating periodization*. It is very similar to what we did at Level 2, only now we will be varying intensity and volume between different weeks instead of different days of the week.

In the first exercise of each training session we will be using my Advanced Training Program (ATP) wave. ATP employs a three-stage microcycle. Your calculations for a particular exercise for one microcycle will be based on the weight you are planning to use in that exercise on the third week. That weight will be considered 100%.

On the first week of a microcycle you perform 5 sets of 6 reps in all strength exercises. The MTLs you use here will be 80% of the weights you are planning to use in those exercises on week three. So simply multiply those weights for each exercise by 0.8.

On the second week you will use 90% of the weights you are planning to use on the third week. So simply multiply those weights by 0.9. You will perform 5 sets of 4 reps with the multiplication products for the respective exercises.

Finally, on the third week you will use the weight that you used as 100% during your previous calculations for a particular exercise and will complete 5 sets of 2 reps with it. Just make sure you are being reasonable when you plan that weight for your very first microcycle. (The same goes for all other parameters of those training sessions).

Successful completion of all prescribed sets and reps in any of the exercises of the microcycle allows you to increase the MTLs in those exercises for the following microcycle. Depending on how comfortable MTL felt for 5x2 in a particular exercise on the third week, you can add 5-10 pounds to it. Now this new MTL will be considered as 100% for this exercise for the new microcycle. Therefore, the MTLs for the first two weeks of this new microcycle will change accordingly.

All of this might sound incredibly complicated but, once you get the idea, it is actually pretty simple. We will use Back Squat to illustrate. Let's say you plan to use 405lbs for your third week. On week one you will use 80% of that MTL:

405 x 0.8 = 324lbs

This means that after proper warm-up you will perform 5 sets of 6 reps with 324lbs. The next time you do Back Squat is on Monday of the following week and you will be using 90% of your third week MTL:

405 x 0.9 = 365lbs

Then on Monday of week 3, you will perform 5 sets of 2 reps with 405. If you were able to complete all the sets and reps in our Squat example, your following three weeks could look like this:

Monday #4 – 5x6 (332lbs)
Monday #5 – 5x4 (373.5lbs)
Monday #6 – 5x2 (415lbs)

During the first two weeks the weight will feel pretty comfortable, but this doesn't mean that you get to relax. Good work done on 5x6 and 5x4 days will ensure successful performance on the following 5x2 days, so make every rep count. Lift the weight as fast as possible during all work sets. Such an explosive style, however, is not an excuse for sloppy form. Only the speed of concentric contraction should increase. All other technical components of exercise execution stay the same.

Not every gym has sets of the very small plates available. Therefore, using exact weights from your calculation might not be possible. No worries. Just round the products of your calculations to the closest weight you can construct. For example, 324 could be rounded to 325. 353 could be rounded to either 352.5 or 355.

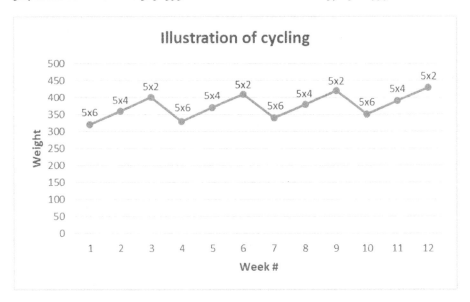

During Level 4 instead of EMOM protocol, we will be utilizing the circuit method. That means that you will not be getting any breaks whatsoever between exercises. These rotations are specifically designed in such a way that there should be a minimum time for transitioning from one exercise to the next, even in a crowded gym.

For example, after you finish the first set of Seated Cable Rows, you will grab a pair of dumbbells (probably slightly heavier than what you used for Shoulder Press during the previous training session) and lay down on the same bench you were just sitting on while rowing. Once you complete Dumbbell Bench Press, you will put one of the dumbbells aside and move on to the Goblet Squats while holding the other dumbbell by your chest with two hands. After that, you put the dumbbell down and go back to the Horizontal Rows right away.

We will also be implementing cyclical variations of intensity and volume for the circuits. During the first week you will perform five rounds of circuits. During the second week you will perform four rounds of circuits while using slightly heavier weights than what you used in the first week. During the third week you will perform three rounds of circuits while using slightly heavier weights than what you used on the second week.

Once the microcycle is completed you can look back at your performance and see if you can increase any weights you are using in the circuits for the following three weeks. Also, remember that on Monday of week 4 you will start with the different circuit from what you did on Monday of week 1.

As far as Back Extensions and Sit-Ups you will continue doing the same thing as you did in Level 3. On the other hand, your running will be quite different. First of all, we will increase the length of each round to 5 minutes (heavier trainees can continue using 3 minutes). Also, the number of rounds and the speed of running will be different between different weeks and different days of the same week.

The reason for that is that once you reach high enough speed it becomes very difficult to maintain it for days and weeks in a row. That is why we will implement a three-week microcycle where you are moving from higher volume and lesser speed to lower volume and higher speed.

Besides decreasing the speed by 1 mph at each following session of the same week similar to the level 3, you will now also decrease the number of rounds by one with each consecutive week of a particular microcycle. At the same time, the speed on all days of the week will increase by 0.5 mph with each successive week of that microcycle. This is what things would look like if 8 mph was my maximum speed:

	MONDAY	WEDNESDAY	FRIDAY
WEEK 1	3X5 (7 mph)	4x5 (6 mph)	5x5 (5 mph)
WEEK 2	2x5 (7.5 mph)	3x5 (6.5 mph)	4x5 (5.5 mph)
WEEK 3	1x5 (8 mph)	2x5 (7 mph)	3x5 (6 mph)

If I was able to complete all the rounds from the example above without overexerting myself, for the following microcycle I would move everything up by 0.1:

	MONDAY	WEDNESDAY	FRIDAY
WEEK 4	3X5 (7.1 mph)	4x5 (6.1 mph)	5x5 (5.1 mph)
WEEK 5	2x5 (7.6 mph)	3x5 (6.6 mph)	4x5 (5.6 mph)
WEEK 6	1x5 (8.1 mph)	2x5 (7.1 mph)	3x5 (6.1 mph)

Hopefully, by now you are starting to recognize the overall theme of Level 4: you push yourself to the limit only one week out of three. The thinking here is that if you have completed all of the previous levels as was prescribed, by now your training sessions have turned into all-out battles. And, in order for you to prevent burning out, these wars have to be interspersed by training with lower intensity.

EXERCISES

Back Extension

Primary movers: spinal erectors.
Secondary movers: gluteus, hamstrings.

Starting position:
- Position the upper portion of your thighs firmly against the pads.
- Hook your heels under the roller pads.
- Keep your arms crossed on your chest.
- Tighten your lower back in a slightly arched position.

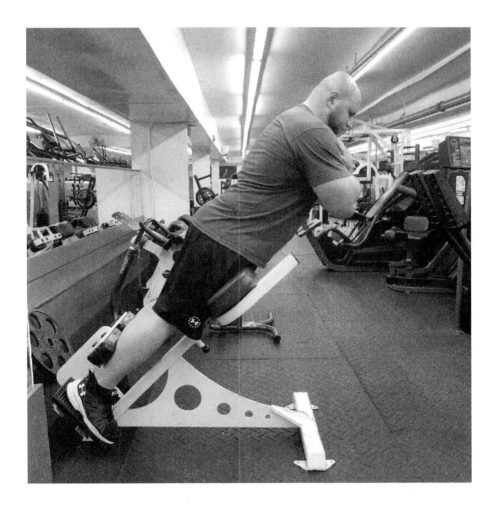

Movement:
- Lower your torso in a controlled manner until it is almost perpendicular to the floor.
- Return to the starting position.

Common mistakes:
- Not going through full ROM.
- Bouncing off from the bottom position.
- Excessive hyperextension at the top position.

Caution:
- Avoid apparatus that place your knees in hyperextension.

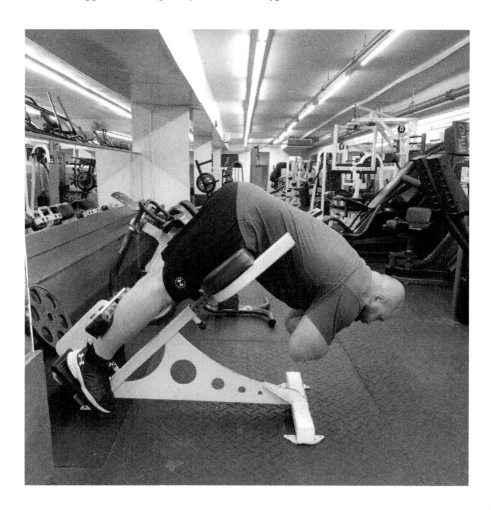

Back Squat

Primary movers: quadriceps, gluteus, hamstrings.
Secondary movers: spinal erectors, adductors, calves.

Starting position:
- Find a comfortable place for the bar on your upper traps (not on your neck).
- Place your hands palms facing forward over the bar slightly wider than your shoulder width (very wide grip makes it difficult to maintain the tightness of the upper back needed to support the bar).
- Place your feet in line about shoulder-width apart.
- Tighten your lower back in slightly arched position and bring your chest up.

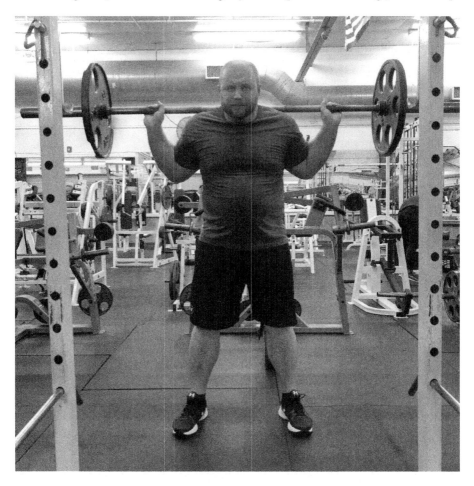

- Unrack the weight while keeping your back tight and take two steps back.
- Position your feet about shoulder-width apart with toes pointing 20-30 degrees out.

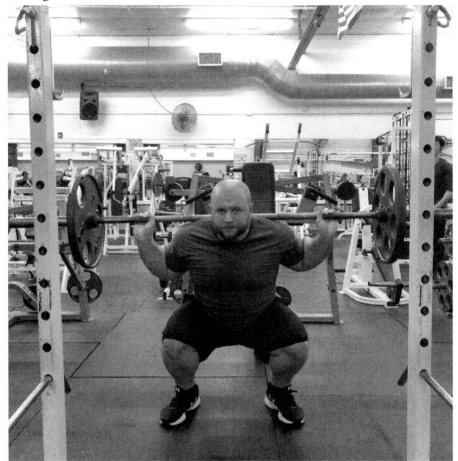

Movement:
- Simultaneously unlock your knees and hips and descend into a position where your thighs are slightly below the parallel level with the floor.
- Do not exaggerate bounce at the bottom position.
- As you are coming up make sure that the extension of hips and knees is happening at the same rate.
- Make sure the center of mass is over the middle of your feet the whole time.
- Maintain a slight arch in your lower back at all times.
- Keep looking forward at the level slightly below your eye level.

- Make sure that your knees point in the same direction as your feet during both descent and ascent.
- Make sure to maintain a tight torso until the bar is returned to the rack.
- Avoid any unnecessary rotation of the torso while moving the bar off and onto the rack.

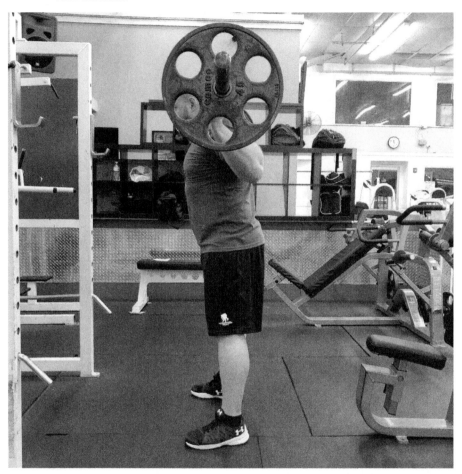

Common mistakes:
- Not descending deep enough (if consistent lack of depth is observed, it might be beneficial to perform Squat with 1-second pause at the bottom during at least some of the warm-up sets).
- Excessive bending at the hips combined with lack of knee flexion (as in Good Morning exercise).
- Shifting center of the mass on heels or towards toes.

- Allowing the knees to move inwards on ascent/descent.
- Rounding your lower back (usually at the bottom – called "butt wink").
- Bouncing from the bottom of the Squat.

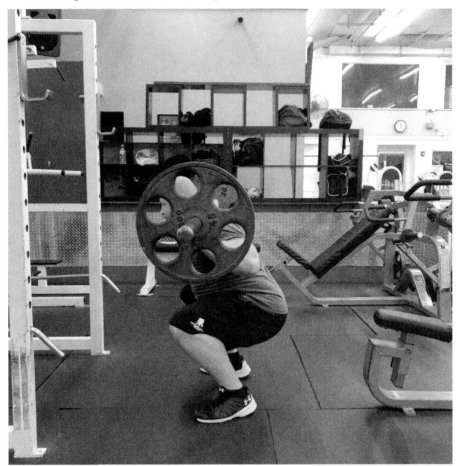

Alternative:
- Low bar position on the back might allow heavier loads to be used but will also shift some emphasis from quadriceps to hip extensors and lower back.

Caution:
- Even when a spotter is present, it is safer to perform Squat inside a power rack or with suspension straps.
- Weightlifting belt could be used for additional back support when very heavy loads are attempted.

Barbell Bench Press

Primary movers: pectorals.
Secondary movers: triceps, anterior deltoids.

Starting position:
- Lie down on your back on a flat bench.
- Slightly arch your lower back and bring your chest up.
- Squeeze your shoulder blades together.
- Place your feet flat on the floor with your knees bent at about 90 degrees.
- Grasp the bar with palms facing towards your legs.
- Select the grip width that will make your forearms parallel to each other (and perpendicular to the bar) at the point when the bar touches your chest.

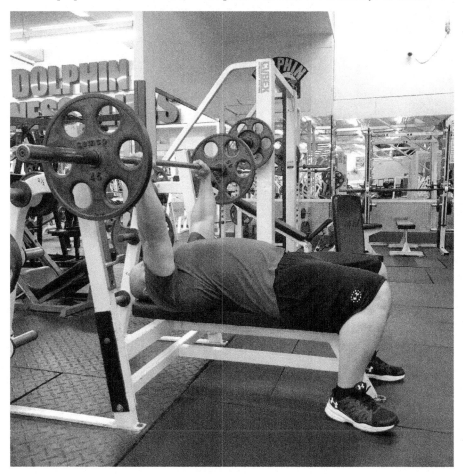

- Position the bar in your hands between head line and life line of your palm with thumbs wrapped around.
- Unrack the bar and position it over your chest on extended arms.

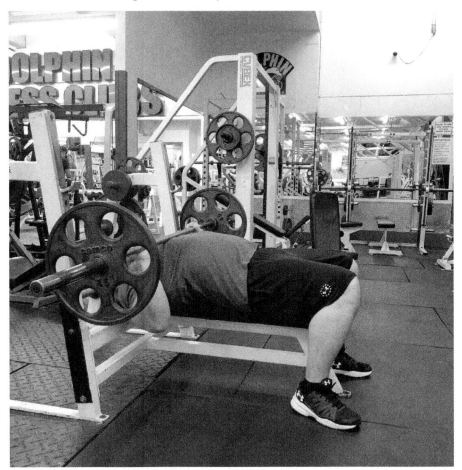

Movement:
- Lower the bar to your chest at about the level of your nipples (the movement will not be strictly vertical but rather a slight arc).
- Once you touch your chest, push it back up in the opposite direction until your arms are straight.
- Maintain elbows under the bar on both descent and ascent.
- Do not attempt to rack the bar until full elbow extension is attained.

Common mistakes:

- Uneven descent/ascent of the bar.
- Allowing your buttocks to come off of the bench at any time.
- Lowering the bar too high on the chest (towards the neck)
- Not lowering the bar all the way to the chest.
- Bouncing the bar off of your chest (if this problem persists, it might be beneficial to perform Bench Press with 1-second pause at the bottom position during at least some of the warm-up sets).
- Not extending your elbows fully at the top of the movement (although hyperextension of elbows must also be avoided).
- Allowing your elbows to flare out excessively to the side.

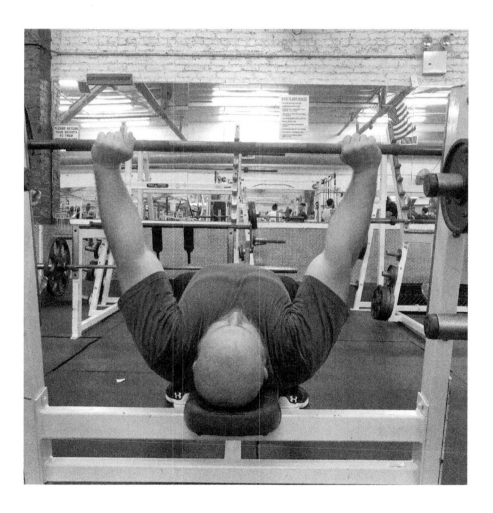

- Excessive wrist extension during movement.
- Using a thumbless grip.

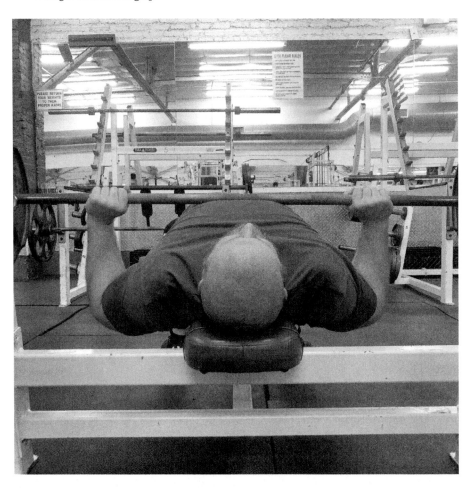

Alternative:
- Excessive arching of lower back reduces the distance the bar has to travel and allows to lift slightly heavier weight. Unless you are preparing for a powerlifting meet, however, this practice is counterproductive as the business at the gym is not about making things easier.

Caution:
- Presence of a spotter is a must when a substantial load is being used.

Deadlift

Primary movers: spinal erectors, gluteus, hamstrings, quadriceps.
Secondary movers: lats, traps.

Starting position:
- Place your feet shoulder-width or slightly narrower with your toes pointing forward (or slightly out).
- Before you bend over to grasp the bar your shins should be about an inch away from it.
- Tighten your lower back in a slightly arched position and maintain it throughout the exercise.

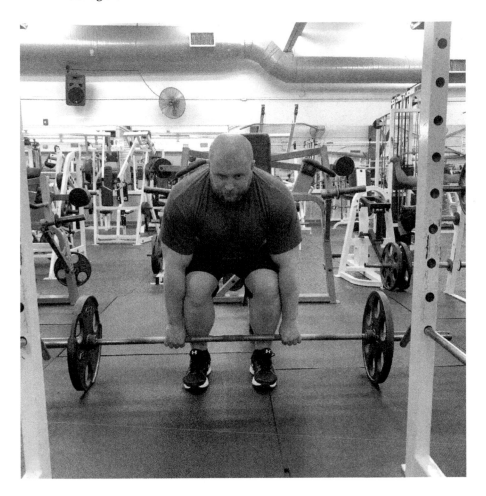

- Squat down to grasp the bar while flexing slightly more at the hips and slightly less at your knees when compared to the Back Squat.
- Grasp the bar with the grip right outside of your legs with palms facing you.
- Keep your chest up and your shoulders slightly in front of the bar.
- Look straight forward.

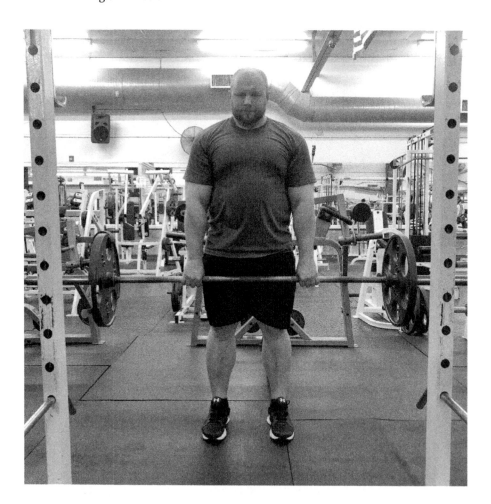

Movement:
- Stand up with the bar held in completely straight arms.
- Make sure the bar stays in contact with your legs the whole time.
- Once the fully upright position is attained, lower the bar back on the floor.

- Make sure that your knees point in the same direction as your feet during both descent and ascent.
- Do not try to bounce the weight off the floor for the following rep.

Common mistakes:
- Rounding your lower back.
- Allowing the knees to move inwards on ascent/descent.
- Allowing the bar to drift away from the front of the legs (usually the result of premature straightening of legs in the beginning of movement).
- Excessive hyperextension at the top.
- Bending of the elbows.

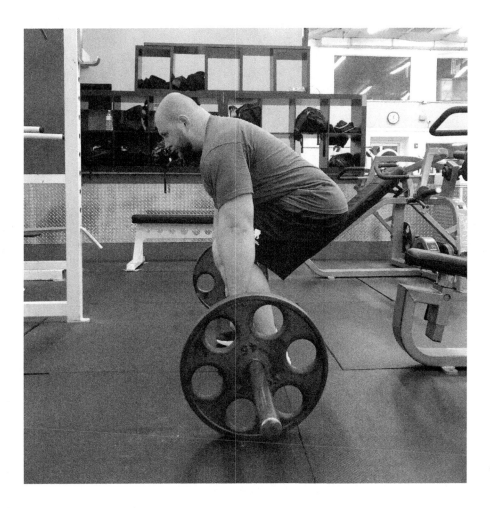

Caution:
- Even though *alternate grip* (one hand supinated, one hand pronated) is often utilized, its use presents an inherent danger. Unless you are planning to compete in a powerlifting contest, use straps when the grip becomes a weak point of the lift.
- Weightlifting belt could be used for additional back support when very heavy loads are attempted.

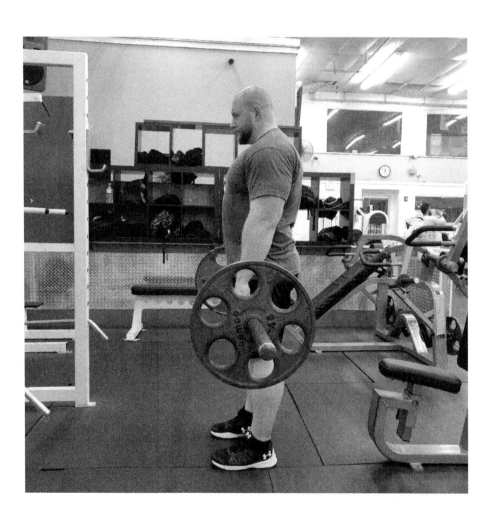

Dumbbell Bench Press

Primary movers: pectorals.
Secondary movers: anterior deltoids, triceps.

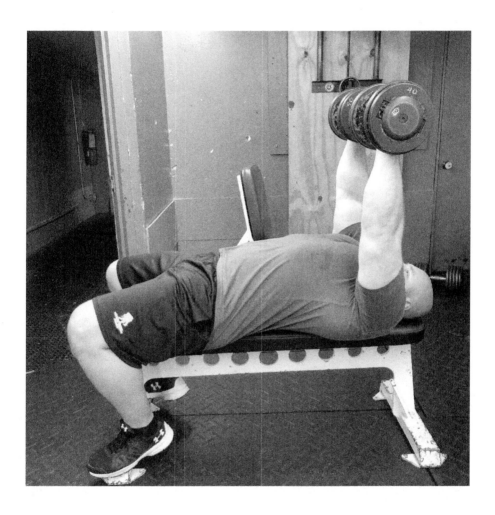

Starting position:
- Lie down on your back on a flat bench.
- Slightly arch your lower back and bring your chest up.
- Squeeze your shoulder blades together.
- Position a pair of dumbbells over your chest on straight arms with palms facing towards your legs (help of a spotter might be needed to get into starting position).

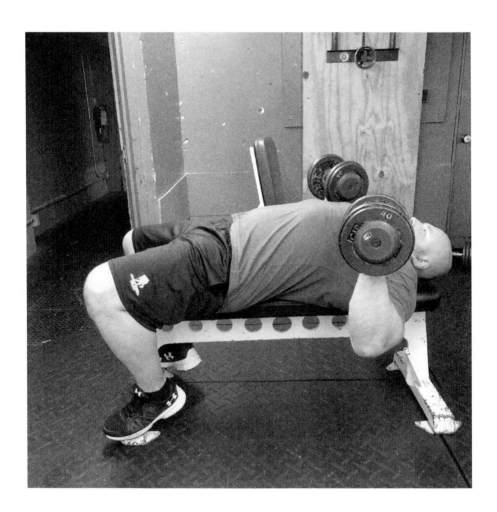

Movement:

- Lower dumbbells to your sides in a wide arc while keeping your forearms parallel to each other.
- Once a comfortable pectoral stretch is attained, push the dumbbells up and together until the arms are straight.

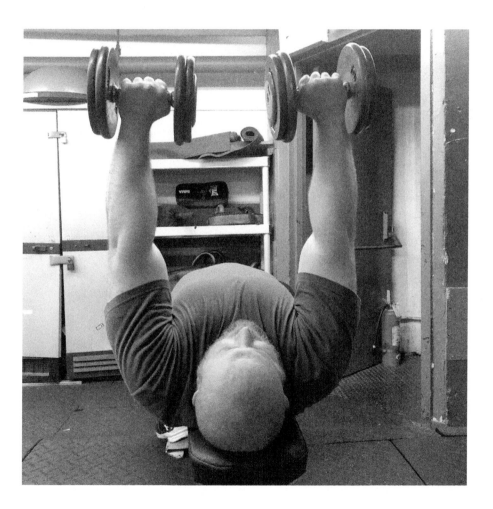

Common mistakes:
- Allowing the buttocks to come off the bench.
- Not going through full ROM.

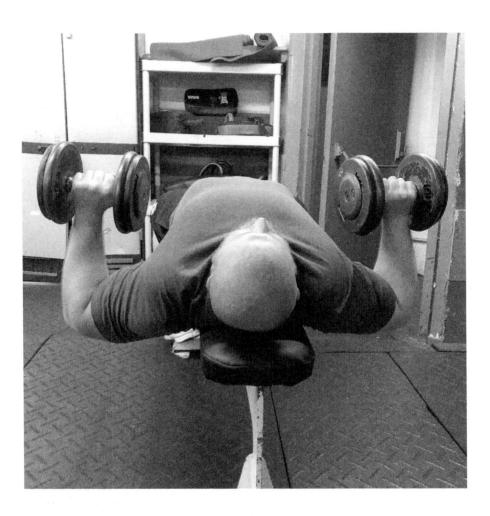

Dumbbell Shoulder Press

Primary movers: anterior and lateral deltoids.
Secondary movers: triceps, traps.

Starting position:
- Sit on the chair with back support (as shown) or stand with your feet shoulder-width apart.
- Keep your chest high and maintain natural arch in your lower back.
- Position dumbbells on the sides of your shoulders at about chin level.
- Palms facing forward but could also be slightly turned in.

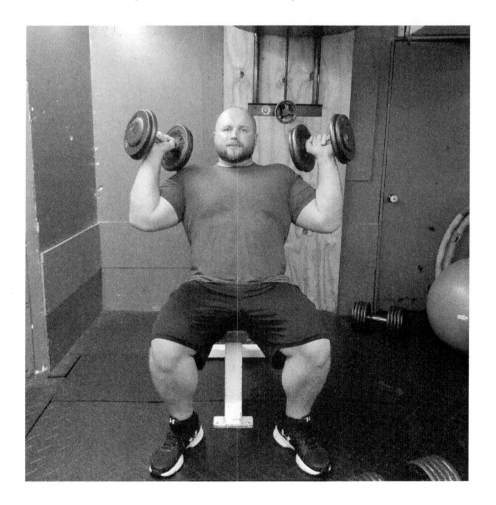

Movement:
- Press the dumbbells up and together over your head until arms are straight.
- Return dumbbells into starting position.

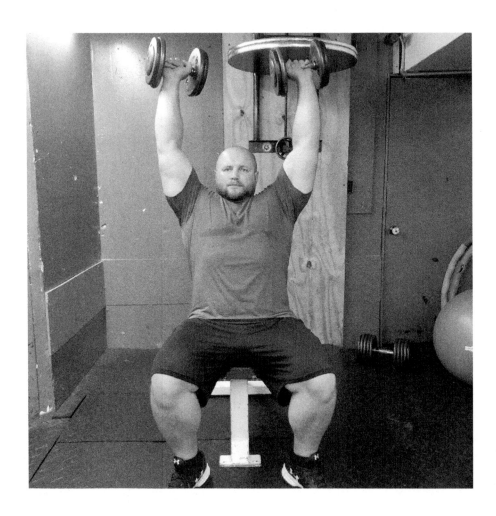

Common mistakes:
- Not going through the full ROM.
- Pressing the dumbbells forward instead of over your head.
- Not maintaining elbows directly under the dumbbells.
- Creating momentum with your legs (in standing version).

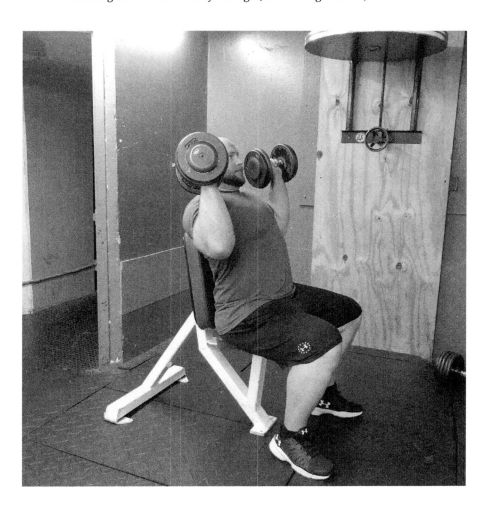

Alternative:
- Although this exercise could also be performed while seated, training programs included in this book prescribe the standing version.

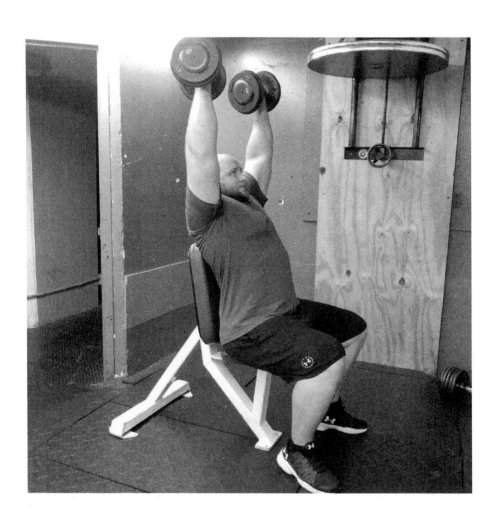

Goblet Squat

Primary movers: quadriceps, gluteus.
Secondary movers: hamstrings, adductors, spinal erectors, calves.

Starting position:
- Position your feet about shoulder-width apart with toes pointing 20-30 degrees out.
- Tighten your lower back in a slightly arched position and bring your chest up.
- Hold a dumbbell with two hands by your chest at the level slightly below your chin.

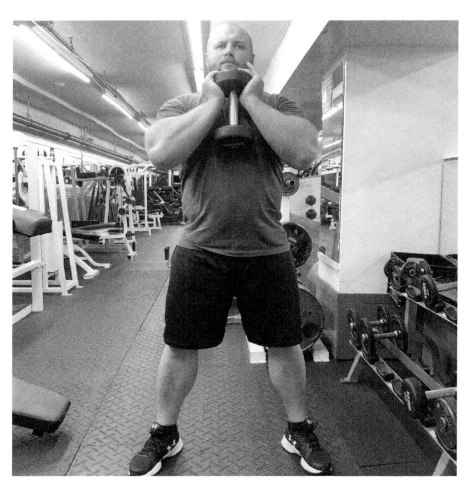

Movement:

- Unlock your knees and descend into a position where your thighs are slightly below the parallel level with the floor while maintaining torso almost vertical.
- Do not exaggerate bounce at the bottom position.
- As you coming up make sure to maintain your torso upright.
- Make sure the center of mass is over the middle of your feet the whole time.
- Maintain a slight arch in your lower back at all times.
- Keep looking forward during both descent and ascent.
- Make sure that your knees point in the same direction as your feet during both descent and ascent.

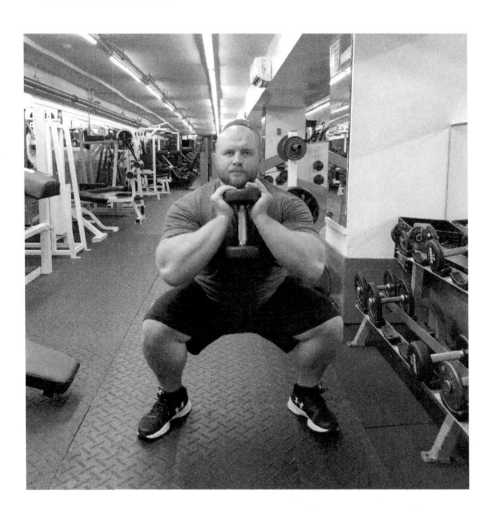

Common mistakes:
- Not descending deep enough.
- Rounding your lower back.
- Failure to maintain upright torso (in this case you might feel that your weight is shifting to the front of your feet).
- Allowing the knees to move inwards on ascent/descent.
- Bouncing from the bottom of the Squat.

Leg Press

Primary movers: quadriceps, gluteus.
Secondary movers: hamstrings, adductors.

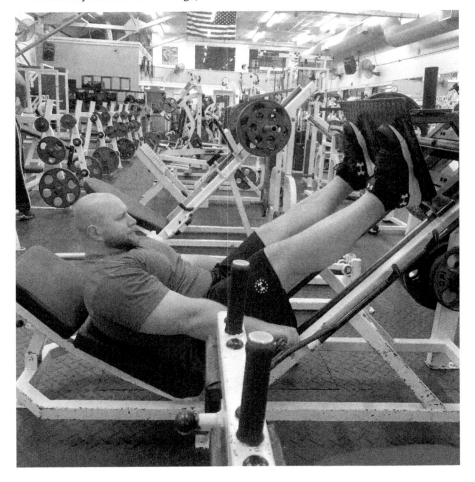

Starting position:

- Position yourself in the seat with your back flat against the pad.
- Place your feet on the platform about shoulder-width apart with your toes pointing slightly out.
- Unrack the weight on the straight (but not hyperextended) legs and remove the supports.

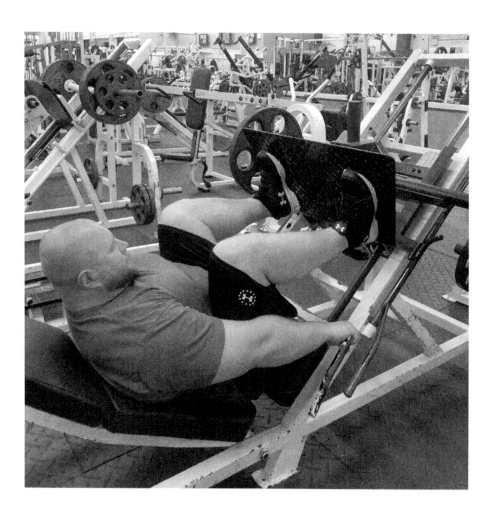

Movement:

- Lower the platform down until your thighs are near the sides of your torso.
- Do not allow your lower back to come off of the seat pad at the bottom position.
- Press the platform back up until your legs are almost straight (never hyperextended).
- Make sure that your knees point in the same direction as your feet during both descent and ascent.
- Make sure to maintain even pressure throughout the soles of your feet.

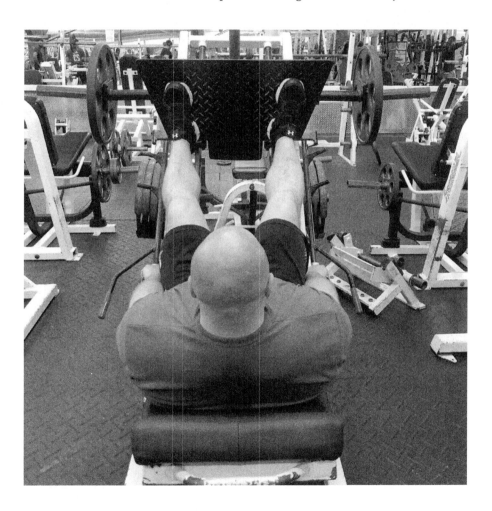

Common mistakes:

- Not going through the full ROM.
- Allowing your lower back to come off of the seat pad (most commonly happens if the feet are positioned too high on the platform).
- Allowing the knees to move inwards on ascent/descent.
- Allowing the heels to come off of the platform at the bottom portion of the movement.

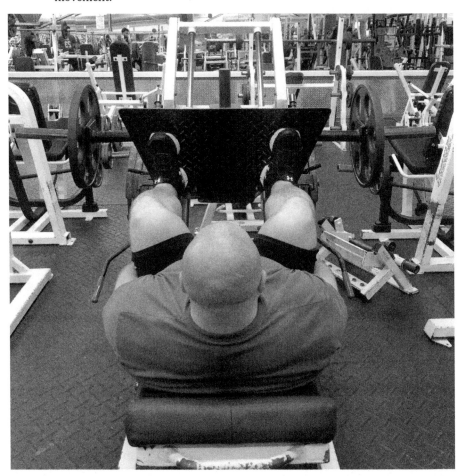

Caution:

- Vertical version of Leg Press makes it very difficult to keep lower back against the seat at the bottom of the movement and should be considered a poor substitute.

Lunge

Primary movers: quadriceps, gluteus, hamstrings.
Secondary movers: adductors, calves.

Starting position:
- Position two dumbbells by your sides with palms facing each other or one dumbbell by your chest at the level slightly below your chin (as in Goblet Squat).
- Make a wide step forward (find a step length at which front leg is just a little past the vertical line at the bottom of the lunge).
- Turn your forward foot slightly inward.

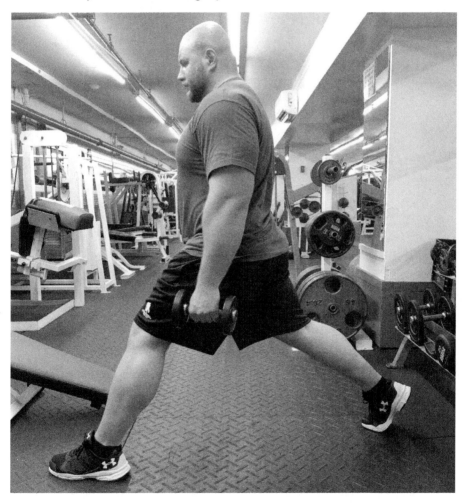

Movement:

- Lower yourself down until the back knee almost touches the floor.
- Bring yourself back up.
- Maintain your torso almost vertical on descent/ascent.
- Make sure your forward knee is aligned with the foot on the descent/ascent.
- Complete all reps on one side before switching to the other leg. It is also possible to perform this exercise in an alternating fashion (while walking forward), but it requires the reset of the starting position on every rep.

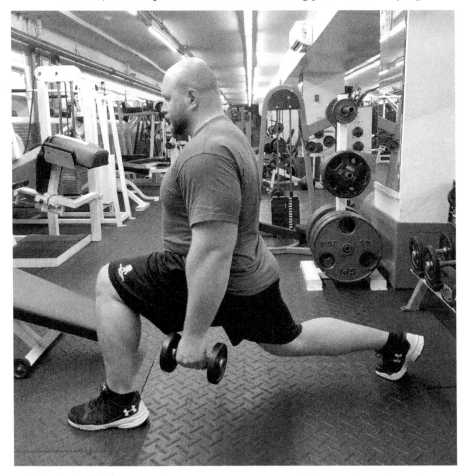

Common mistakes:

- Positioning front foot straight forward.
- Not lowering down enough (might be due to lack of flexibility).
- Allowing the forward knee to go past the toes at the bottom position.

Pulldown

Primary movers: lats.
Secondary movers: biceps, posterior deltoids.

Starting position:
- Sit on the seat and hook your thighs under the roller pads.
- Grasp the bar shoulder-width or wider with your palms facing forward.
- Allow your shoulder blades to come slightly out and up.
- Your arms should be straight with the bar directly over your head.

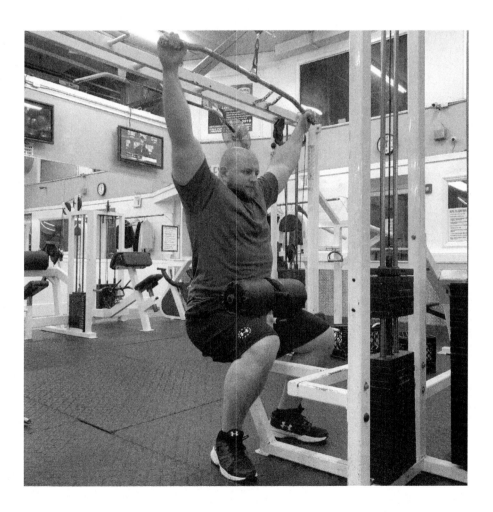

Movement:
- Pull the bar down to your chest while simultaneously raising your chest up.
- Lean back a little during the descent to allow the bar to go past your face.
- Touch your chest with the bar while simultaneously squeezing your shoulder blades together.
- Return the bar back onto outstretched arms.

Common mistakes:
- Not going through full ROM (usually means that the weight is too heavy).
- Creating momentum with explosive back extension.
- Not allowing shoulder blades to come out at the top.
- Not squeezing your shoulder blades together at the bottom.

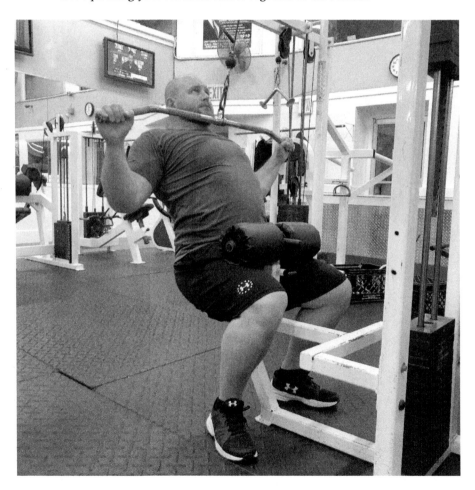

Seated Cable Row

Primary movers: lats.
Secondary movers: spinal erectors, biceps, posterior deltoids, traps.

Starting position:
- Sit on the seat with your feet positioned on the platform in front of you.
- Tighten your lower back in a slightly arched position.
- Bend your knees slightly and maintain that position the whole time.
- Hold the parallel handles with palms facing each other.
- Keep your arms straight and allow your shoulder blades to move slightly out.

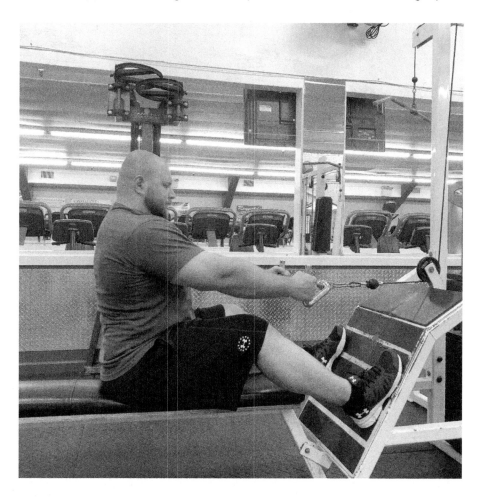

Movement:
- Pull the handles into your belly while sliding your elbows against your ribs.
- Keep your chest up and squeeze your shoulder blades together at the end of the pull.
- Return the weight to the starting position.
- It is natural if your torso moves slightly forward at the beginning of the pull and slightly back at the end of it.

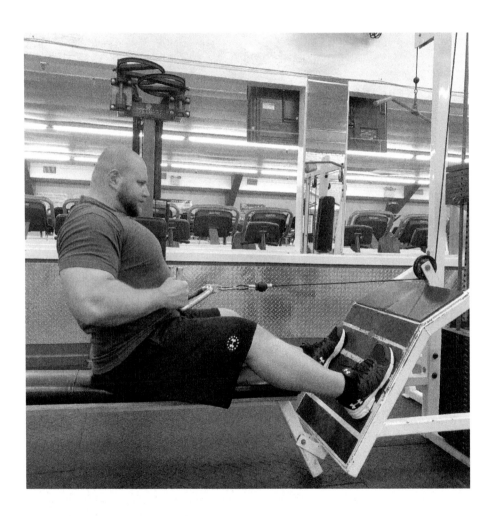

Common mistakes:
- Pulling of the weight towards the chest instead of the abdomen.
- Not going through full ROM (usually means that the weight is too heavy).
- Creating momentum with explosive back extension.
- Not allowing shoulder blades to come out in the beginning of the pull.
- Not squeezing your shoulder blades together at the end of the pull.
- Rounding your lower back.

Sit-Up

Primary movers: abdominals.
Secondary movers: hip flexors.

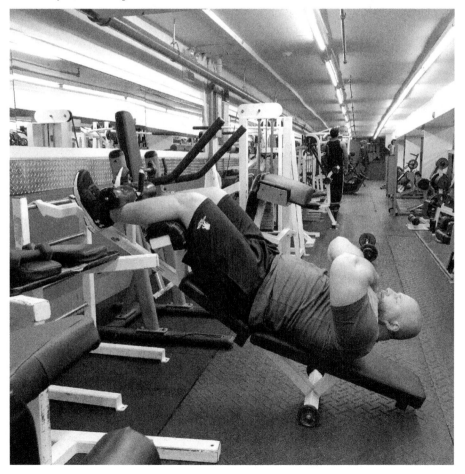

Starting position:
- Hook your feet under the roller pads.
- Lie down on the incline bench with your head down (the higher your legs in relation to the head, the more difficult the exercise will be).
- Tuck your chin down to your chest.
- Cross your arms on your chest with your fingers touching your shoulders (unless you are holding a plate on your chest).

Movement:
- Curl your torso up and touch the lower portions of your thighs with your elbows.
- Return to the starting position.

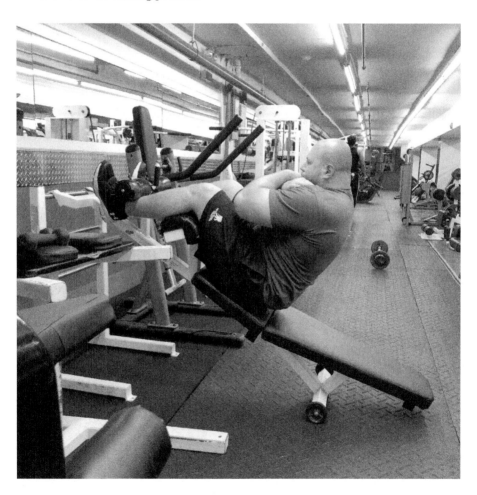

Common mistakes:
- Not keeping your hands in contact with the shoulders (if you are holding a plate, keep it close to your chin).
- Pulling on your head during ascent.
- Performing the ascent in ballistic fashion.
- Keeping the torso very rigid (will make hip flexors do most of the work).

Alternative:
- Out of shape beginners might need to start with Crunches (shown below) and switch to Sit-Ups few months later.

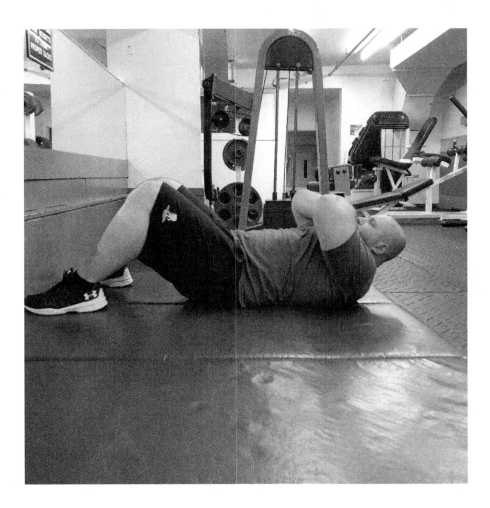

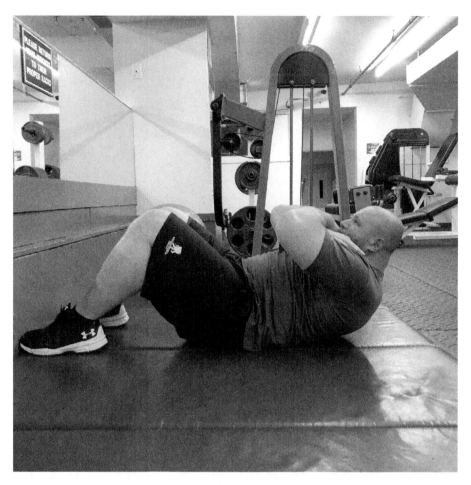

- While keeping your lower back on the mat, curl your torso towards the legs (another way to think about Crunches is as trying to pinch your ribs and pelvis together).
- Squeeze your abdominals at the top for a moment and return to the starting position.

Stretching

Muscles stretched: pectorals.

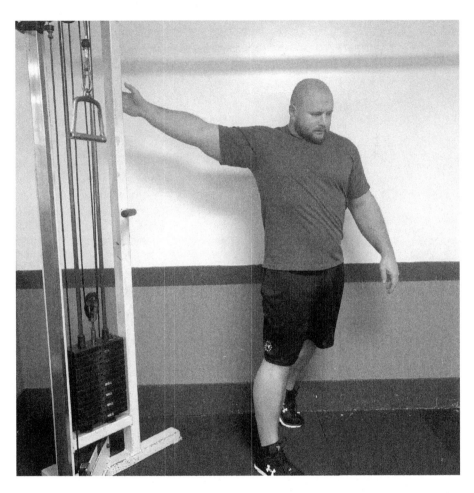

- Grab a stable object (as shown in the picture above) slightly higher than the shoulder level.
- Lean forward while also turning slightly away from the object.

Muscles stretched: upper back.

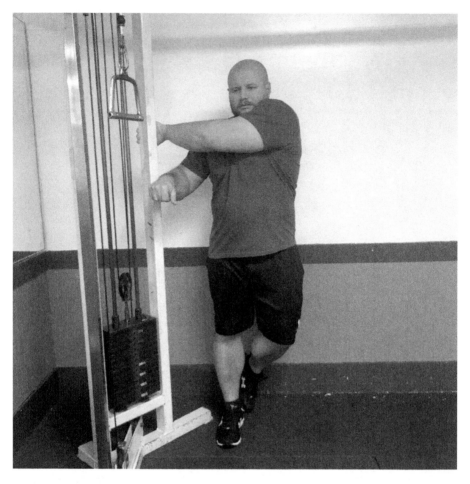

- Grab a stable object (as shown in the picture above) at about the level of your shoulders.
- Lean to the opposite side from the object while also turning slightly away from it.

Muscles stretched: lats.

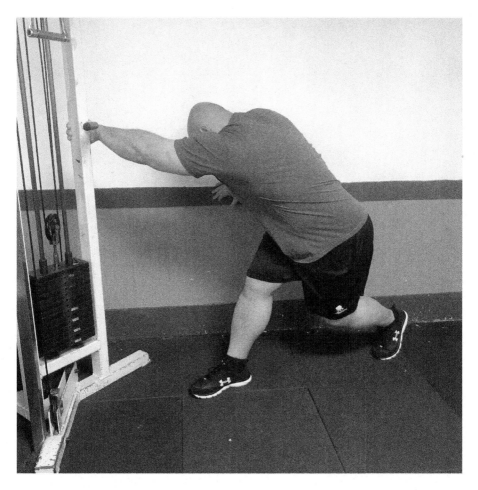

- Grab a stable object (as shown in the picture above) at the level somewhere between your shoulders and waist.
- Shift your bodyweight back while also turning ipsilateral hip away from the outstretched arm.

Muscles stretched: traps.

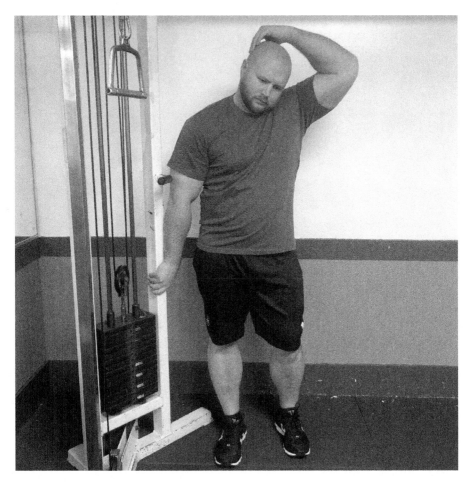

- Grab a stable object (as shown in the picture above) at the level that creates taut traps on the same side.
- Lean slightly to the opposite side from the object while also tilting your head away from it.
- You can also apply very light pressure on the head with your fingers (as shown in the picture), as long as it does not create any neck discomfort.

Muscles stretched: quadriceps.

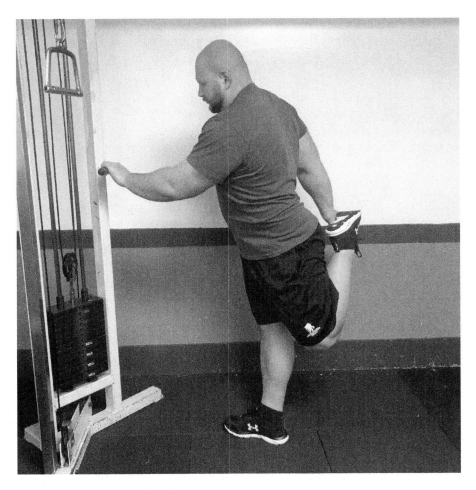

- Grab a stable object for balance.
- Grab a foot with the contralateral arm (as shown in the picture above).
- Bring the foot of the leg that is being stretched to the ipsilateral glute.
- While keeping the knee fully flexed, pull the thigh slightly back.
- Make sure not to lean forward as you are pulling the thigh back.

Muscles stretched: calves.

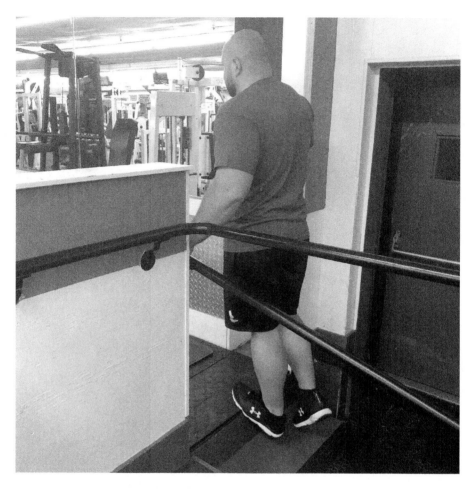

- Position the ball of one foot on the edge of a step.
- While keeping the leg straight, lower the heel of the same foot down until a comfortable calf stretch is attained.

Muscles stretched: hamstrings and lower back.

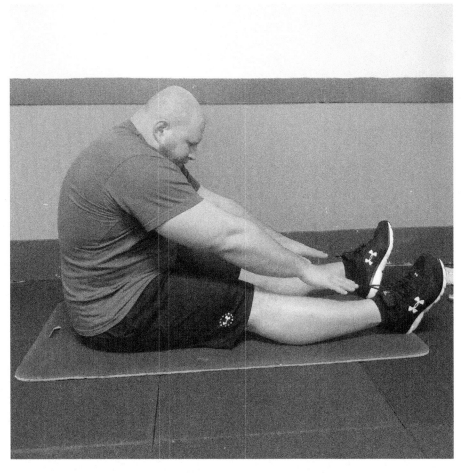

- Sit on the floor with your legs extended (or slightly bent if the straight position creates significant knee discomfort).
- Lean forward towards your feet (as shown in the picture above).
- You can also gently pull yourself forward while holding on to your feet or ankles with your hands.

NUTRITION

FIT IN ONE YEAR

The information presented in this chapter is meant to give you a general outline of nutritional intake. Practical applications, however, will vary greatly depending on the particular circumstances of each individual. That is why it is imperative to consult your physician before implementing any recommendations presented here.

There is a lot of confusion on this topic and l will try not to add to it. It seems that common sense becomes less and less common when it comes to nutrition. In theory, we could calculate how many grams of each macronutrient we need. Make sure everything is organic and gluten-free. Plus don't forget about eliminating all the bad cholesterol, of course.

The more practical approach is to take your current diet and try to improve it over time. Making small changes is the key here. Anything too radical will most likely not last very long. Oftentimes people attempt diets that nobody could possibly sustain and then end up quitting in a matter of days. "At least I tried." Instead, let's talk about how to actually make it work this time.

Meal schedule

We will start with the meal schedule. Ideally, you should be eating 4-6 times a day with your meals evenly spread out. Generally, the smaller and leaner your meals are the more of them you will be able to squeeze in one day (large fatty meals will sit in your stomach longer). Also, try not to lie down right after meals. Instead, take a short walk to expedite the emptying of the stomach.

If you currently eat three times a day, try to have a snack somewhere. It is really not that hard and a very busy schedule is no excuse. For instance, if there is a long gap between your breakfast and lunch, just add an apple and a handful of almonds somewhere in between. Don't change too many things at once and give your body time to adjust. You can't go overnight from eating three times a day to eating eight. Just like you can't jump from squatting 300 pounds to squatting 800.

We all know that breakfast is the most important meal. It fuels you for the rest of the day. There is one more important meal though. It is thought that immediately after training sessions our metabolism is in its heightened state and the ability of muscle tissue to uptake nutrients is increased. This window is considered to be open for about an hour and it would be wise to have a quality meal within this time.

One more thing you have to take into account when spacing your meals throughout the day is your pre-workout meal timing. A lot of it is a matter of personal preference. In general, after a large meal you should allow about three hours before hitting the gym, after a medium-size meal – two hours and after a small meal – about an hour. Try to avoid anything with a lot of fat or fiber at this time as this will slow the digestion and might make you feel bloated during the following training session.

Calories

Calories are used to measure the amount of energy we receive from consuming one gram of a *macronutrient*. The latter includes protein, carbohydrates (carbs) and fats. One gram of protein or carbs has 4 calories. One gram of fat has 9. Such a difference in energy density is one of the reasons to keep the consumption of fats under control when dieting.

Whether you are trying to gain muscle mass or to lose body fat the principles of proper nutritional intake will remain the same. The only difference is that when the goal is to gain muscle you have to consume more calories than you spend and when the goal is to lose fat you have to consume less than you spend.

Protein

Besides feeding yourself consistently throughout the day make sure to get some protein with every meal. *Amino acids* derived from protein are considered to be the primary medium for muscle tissue synthesis. Therefore, you want to have at least some amount of them circulating in your bloodstream at all times. The best sources of complete protein are eggs, beef, pork, milk (if tolerated), chicken and fish. Those who prefer not to ingest animal products, must be very diligent about making sure you receive a full profile of essential amino acids. If the budget allows, you can also utilize protein supplements. But don't overvalue their benefits. They are just convenient to use sometimes. For example, if your gym is far from your house and you are unable to have a meal within an hour after your workout, a protein shake could be the answer.

Carbs

Carb overview will be a little more extensive. Not because they are more important than other macronutrients, but because a few basic concepts need to be understood in their regard. As always, we will simplify things a little and this quick overview is not meant to turn you into a Registered Dietitian.

Carbs are your primary fuel source. Once a meal rich in carbs has been consumed, they are broken down and absorbed into the bloodstream as *glucose.* The rate at which this process occurs depends on the type of carbs your meal contains. In general, all carbohydrates can be roughly divided into fast absorption (simple) carbs and slow absorption (complex) carbs. The term Glycemic Index (GI) is also commonly used. The higher GI is the faster the absorption will occur. That means that simple carbs have a high GI and complex carbs have a low GI.

Our bodies always try to maintain a certain steady concentration of glucose in the blood. If the blood glucose levels were allowed to drop very low, there wouldn't be an energy source readily available for utilization. If the levels were allowed to rise too high, the blood would start to resemble maple syrup which would impede circulation.

We are now going to take a look at what happens when you consume a meal full of simple carbs (candy, soda, pastries, etc.) versus a meal consisting of mostly complex carbs (pasta, rice, potatoes, oatmeal and yams). Let's say one day you decided to have some donuts and soda for breakfast (point A).

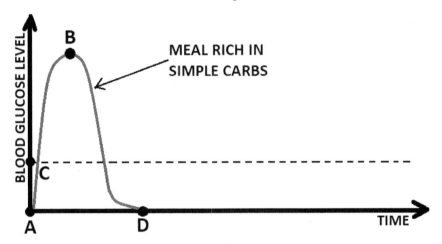

Since your breakfast choices consist of mostly simple carbs, they will be absorbed very quickly and result in a steep increase of the blood glucose level (point B). This will trigger a significant release of insulin in order to bring the blood glucose level down to a desirable level (dotted line C). All excess sugar will be removed from the circulation and stored away to be utilized later.

There are two places where the excess of glucose can be stored. Limited amount of it can be deposited in muscles and liver in a form of *glycogen*. The rest will be converted to fat and stored in adipose tissue. If you have been to any American metropolis lately, you already know that the capacity of that reservoir is virtually unlimited.

Depending on the size of your breakfast, all this might happen in an hour or two. But now let's imagine that you have 4 hours between breakfast and lunch (point D). Where are you going to get the energy for the other two hours? Those who have been paying attention so far will answer: from stored glycogen and body fat. That is a partially correct answer. Good job! Bear in mind, however, that when our body is in starvation mode it will also tap into muscle tissue as a source of energy. Such catabolic process is obviously not desirable. Also, since you will be essentially fasting from this point, the feeling of low energy and fatigue will accompany that time period.

The situation will be different if you eat a bowl of oatmeal for breakfast. Oatmeal is a complex carb and will be digested slowly. This means that you will have a steady source of energy for longer. It also means that you will avoid storing body fat (when blood glucose is too high) and tapping into muscle tissues for energy (when blood glucose is too low).

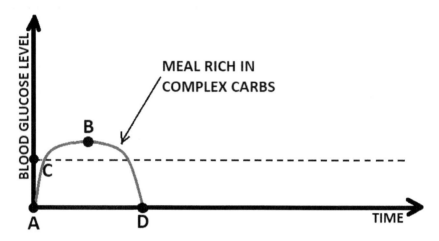

Hopefully, the above comparison of how different types of carbs get utilized made it clear that any extreme fluctuations of the blood glucose level are undesirable. For that reason, it is also generally recommended that instead of large seldom meals, athletes consume smaller but more frequent meals (A, B, C, D, E on the picture below). Such eating practice will also give you a chance to maintain a steady intake of protein throughout the day.

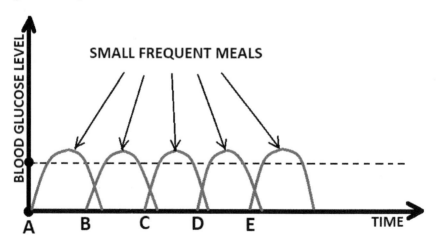

Carb consumption differs from the consumption of protein though. When it comes to protein you generally want to keep its intake even throughout the day. With carbs, on the other hand, try to get more of them earlier in the day and gradually decrease their consumption as the day goes on. This is due to the fact that carbs consumed later in the day will have a smaller chance of being utilized for energy and a higher chance of being stored as fat (some of them will be absorbed when you are already in bed). To illustrate, have eggs with a large portion of oatmeal for breakfast, steak with a moderate amount of potatoes for lunch and chicken with a small amount of rice for dinner. Your late evening snack could be completely carb-free – cottage cheese or Greek yogurt could do the trick.

There are two exceptions here: both pre- and post-workout meals should contain carbs combined with some protein in them, even if you train late in the evening. Carbs consumed before training will provide you with energy for a workout. Carbs consumed afterward will help with recovery. Immediately after a training session is also the time when you should choose eating simple carbs (sports drink, for example) over complex carbs to jumpstart replenishing of glycogen used up during your workout. At other times try to stay away from simple carbs. Soda and other sugary drinks are frequent offenders in this category.

Fats

When it comes to fat you don't need to worry about getting enough of it. Most common diets will provide fat in excess. Therefore, your effort should be directed towards keeping the amount of fat consumed under control. Once again, common sense applies. Reduction of fats below a reasonable level is not only unnecessary but could also be unhealthy. If your diet is full of junk food (pizza, fries, chips), you have some work to do. But as long as you stick to the staple foods mentioned earlier for most of your meals, you should be on the right track.

Water

Among the factors that will determine the amount of water you need are local climate and your activity level. A simple way to monitor your hydration status is by checking the color of your urine. If it's dark and brown – start drinking more. Just keep in mind that some foods and medications could also affect the color of your urine.

Besides drinking with meals, good times to add more water are upon awakening, half an hour before meals and before/during/after training sessions. Don't dive at the deep end right away. Start adding little by little and keep watching the color of your urine. Once it consistently has a clear, pale yellow color you know you found the right amount of water you need.

Fiber

Most of us have an idea of what eating healthy means. Eating lots of fresh fruits and vegetables is always a good policy. Besides being rich in *micronutrients* (vitamins and minerals), fruits and vegetables are an important source of fiber. One of the many benefits of dietary fiber is that it makes your gastrointestinal tract work more efficiently. This is a huge aid when you are trying to get enough nutrients while trying to recover from grueling training sessions. As always, there is no need for anything extreme. Putting away massive amounts of broccoli and asparagus every day will not make you live forever. Instead, it will fill your belly with gas and discomfort.

Supplements

There is a lot of garbage in this industry and it is important to be cautious while navigating it. Your number one concern is safety. Do not take any substances that fall into the dietary supplement category without consulting a qualified healthcare professional. The second factor you should consider is your budget. Remember, supplements are meant to complement a good diet and not to compensate for a bad one. It doesn't make any sense to spend so much money on supplements that now you can't afford real food.

Start with basics. I mentioned protein powder earlier. Also, taking multivitamins and multiminerals with breakfast can help with covering your micronutrients. Creatine is another effective supplement that has been around for some time. Personally, I would always stick to the minimum recommended doses. Plus be especially diligent about staying hydrated if you decide to take it. Aside from this short list, make sure to do research before spending money on a new "ultimate" pill endorsed by some celebrity athlete. The chances are that athlete has never taken it.

Consistency

Just like with training, an effective diet is all about consistency. Anyone can eat clean for a day or even a week. But what you think is going to happen when you return to your normal eating patterns? You are not the first person in the world who wants results as quickly as possible. If there was an easy way to get things done, it would be included in this book.

Hence, abandon the mindset of a temporary fix and start moving towards developing lifelong healthy eating habits. As I stated earlier, don't attempt to adjust your whole diet all at once. Instead, try improving one meal at a time. Making sure you eat proper breakfast is always a good start. Once that's up to standards, you can move on to the next step. When it comes to nutrition, there is always room for improvement. Similarly to how your training will be more complex over time, your diet will have to become more refined as you keep advancing.

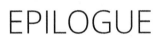

EPILOGUE

Once you have completed all the levels, you will have many options available. You might find yourself interested in joining a local MMA academy or maybe signing up for a "Spartan" race. You could also return to whatever level you liked the most and just focus on maintenance. Don't feel obligated to push yourself to the limit all the time. As long as you keep yourself in decent shape with Level 1 or Level 2 programs, you will be able to step things up at any time.

If you do decide to continue pushing forward, some adjustments might be warranted to prevent burnout and overuse injuries. It could be accomplished by combining three Level 4 microcycles into one macrocycle. This way you wouldn't try to hit a new personal record (PR) every 3 weeks, but instead would work up to it over three consecutive waves.

Let's say you completed 405 pounds in Deadlift for 5x2. Instead of trying to beat it in three weeks, you would deload and then work up to a new PR over nine weeks: 390 for 5x2 on week 3, 400 for 5x2 on week 6, 410 for 5x2 on week 9. After that, you would deload again and then work your way up to 415 during the following 9 weeks. Similar modifications would be implemented for all other elements of training sessions. Just be ready to put the clutch in fifth gear. This is Level 5 – the black belt club!

Those who fell in love with heavy weights I invite to check out my book "Big and Strong Without Steroids." It is a more comprehensive source of information about resistance training intended to give you much deeper understanding of this topic. It also contains multiple complete training programs that can help you with further strength development.

At this point, you have earned your right to get creative. Want to try the rowing machine instead of running? Go right ahead. Thinking about substituting Sit-Ups with Plank? Why not? By now you have learned that the gym is not a playground and you are here to get better. You know that having fun at the gym is not about doing whatever you want. It's about getting the results that you want.

There will always be people for whom nothing that I have said in this book will ever make any sense. Some people are simply addicted to comfort. "Why put yourself through all that?" When I tell them how some of my most memorable moments have happened during combat and fighting - they think that I am out of my mind. Anything that could potentially shorten your lifespan is considered total insanity. Yet wasting year after year of your life just going through the motions is completely acceptable.

Needless to say, I see it differently. I believe that it's all about making your life as adventurous as possible. At the end of the day, both ups and downs make interesting memories. But the only way to truly enjoy such a ride is if you have your mind and your body ready for it. Hopefully, this book can help some of you with that. So enough talking my friends. Let's get to work!

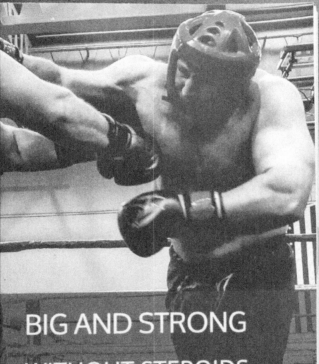

BIG AND STRONG

WITHOUT STEROIDS

Yuriy Oliynyk

Printed in Great Britain
by Amazon

80254888R00058